LOSE WEIGHT EVERYDAY

Yes, You Can & You Will
LOSE WEIGHT EVERYDAY

Using Any Of These
Eleven *NATURAL*
Appetite-control
Products &
Supplements
(Acronymed *NAPS*).

DISCLAIMER AND TERMS OF USE AGREEMENT

Lose Weight Everyday author and publisher have used their best efforts in preparing this Book. The author and publisher make no representation or warranties with respect to the accuracy, applicability, fitness, or completeness of the contents of this Book. **The information is strictly for educational purposes only and is not intended to diagnose, treat, prescribe, prevent or heal any medical disorders. We cannot promise that you will make the same income others have made selling these product**s. Therefore, if you wish to apply the ideas contained in this Book, you are taking full responsibility for your actions, experience and results.

EVERY EFFORT HAS BEEN MADE TO ACCURATELY REPRESENT THESE PRODUCTS AND THEIR POTENTIALS. HOWEVER, THERE IS NO GUARANTEE THAT YOU WILL IMPROVE IN ANY WAY USING NAPS, THE TECHNIQUES OR IDEAS IN THESE MATERIALS. EXAMPLES IN THESE MATERIALS ARE NOT TO BE INTERPRETED AS A PROMISE OR GUARANTEE OF ANYTHING. SELF-HELP AND IMPROVEMENT POTENTIAL ARE ENTIRELY DEPENDENT ON THE PERSON USING THESE PRODUCTS, IDEAS AND TECHNIQUES.

YOUR LEVEL OF IMPROVEMENT IN ATTAINING THE RESULTS CLAIMED IN OUR MATERIALS WILL TOTALLY DEPEND ON YOU. FIRST, ON THE AMOUNT OF TIME YOU DEVOTE TO THE PROGRAM, IDEAS AND TECHNIQUES MENTIONED. SECOND, YOUR WILLINGNESS TO APPLY THE KNOWLEDGE AND VARIOUS SKILLS. SINCE THESE FACTORS DIFFER PER INDIVIDUAL, YOU WILL ACHIEVE ABUNDANTLY OR FAIL MISERABLY. WE CANNOT GUARANTEE YOUR SUCCESS OR IMPROVEMENT LEVEL. NOR ARE WE RESPONSIBLE FOR ANY OF YOUR ACTIONS. SO, TO EXPERIENCE SUCCESS, YOU MUST TAKE DAILY, BOLD, CONSISTENT ACTIONS. TRUST GOD.

MANY FACTORS WILL BE IMPORTANT IN DETERMINING YOUR ACTUAL RESULTS AND NO GUARANTEES ARE MADE THAT YOU WILL ACHIEVE RESULTS LIKE ANYBODY MENTIONED IN THIS BOOK. IN FACT, NO GUARANTEES ARE MADE THAT YOU WILL ACHIEVE ANY RESULTS FROM OUR IDEAS OR TECHNIQUES IN THIS BOOK.

MANY INDIVIDUALS HAVE VERBALISED RESULTS OF VARYING DEGREE AFTER CONSISTENT APPLICATIONS, MAYBE, YOU COULD TOO. SO, BEFORE YOU SAY YOU CAN'T LOSE WEIGHT OR ACHIEVE BIG SUCCESS IN ANYTHING; I SAY BELIEVE IN GOD, ACRONYMED BIG. LIVE UNDER CHRIST KNOWLEGEG, ACRONYMED LUCK. TO THE OBESED, USE NATURAL APPETITE-CONTROL PRODUCTS & SUPPLEMENTS – ACRONYMED NAPS.

The author and publisher disclaim any warranties (express or implied), merchantability, or fitness for any purpose. **The author and publisher shall in no event be held liable to any party for any direct, indirect, punitive, special, incidental or other consequential damages arising directly or indirectly from any use of this material, which is provided "as is", and without warranties.**

The author and publisher disclaim any warranties (express or implied). We do not diagnose, prevent, treat, cure or claim to heal any diseases and as such, respectfully states as always, that you seek the advice of a competent professional healthcare provider before making any changes in your treatment modality.

The author and publisher do not warrant the performance, effectiveness or applicability of any sites listed or linked to in this book.

All links are for information purposes only and are not warranted for content, accuracy or any other implied or explicit purpose. All CPTG Certified Pure Therapeutic Grade Essential Oils and or oil products are products of dōTERRA International and all rights are reserved by them. The author is an affiliate with the company and regular user of their CPTG products with amazing success. Discovering the benefits of their products will depend on your personal uses.

The Lose Weight Team
Upper Marlboro, MD, USA

Websites
1. **Buy Products:** http://bit.ly/2IEZ8V5
2. **For Motivation to Lose Weight Blogsite:**
   http://lose-weight-everyday.com/

Email: contact@lose-weight-everyday.com

TABLE OF CONTENTS

PREFACE

Whatever brought you here, welcome!

"LOSE WEIGHT EVERYDAY" has become one of the biggest challenges that the overweight or obese person is faced with today. Too often, some of these people define themselves by their bulging figure and not their fantastic character. Their self-esteem is decreased because of some negative things some unkind people said about them in the past, and not by the nice things they do everyday for others. So, instead of believing what God said about them in Jermiah 29:11, "*For I know the thoughts that I think toward you, says the LORD, thoughts of peace and not of evil, to give you a future and a hope;*"; they believed the lies of foolish unkind people. Instead of embracing the wonderful instructions from God, such as 1Peter 5:7 which said, "*Cast all your cares upon me, for I care for you*", they train their taste buds to help them cope by craving sugar, salt and fats.

The pleasurable sensation felt when people digest these foods does not last long or help to resolve their insecurities. Sadly, some people increased their intake of this kind of food and lack of frequent exercise, leading many to overweight or obesity.

I invite you, dear overweight or obese reader, to "Believe in God"—acronymed, BIG. You can lose weight in a big way and never regain it. But you must believe you can do it. You are God's created special being and you have everything you need to succeed in a big way at anything, any day in this lifetime. You can do it and you will, just trust God to lead and guide you. He is standing nearby you. You must ask His help though. Believe what He says by reading His Holy Word. Do what the word says.

Here's the truth, I don't know who you are: overweight or obese. I do not care where you are from but I do know one thing; **if you are overweight or obese and decides to use the Natural Appetite-control Products & Supplements - NAPS, embrace the LUCK system we bring to you in this book, and particiapate in our "30-Day Lose Weight Everyday Plan" via your email, you will come out a slimmer, healthier, happier person.**

You can lose weight using our systems. Our systems show the two weights...

1. **Physical weight** made of fat that clogs your arteries causing heart attacks.

2. **The emotional weights** that messes up your mind with anger, hurts, sadness, procrastinations, and so much more. You can believe the lies of unkind people, such as you cannot lose weight, or you will never amount to anything good. You are not a winner et cetera. Instead, you can believe God and start to live your life under that knowledge.

Are you taking out your discouragments on sugary, salty and fatty foods? If so, these substances may make you feel good for a moment (but leave you empty, embarrased, and hiding in big clothes) for a lifetime. That feeling is only the addiction which does not resolve your problems. There will be many complications arising from the addiction, overweight and obesity. Things such as lifestyle diseases, poverty, sadness, depression, poor self-esteem, diabetes, heart failure and so much more.

"Governments worldwide spent over 6 trillion dollars yearly on global healthcare treatments" per the World Health Organization (WHO). Why are people getting sicker from lifestyle diseases when so much money is been spent on treatments? Overweight and obesity are predicted to become a pandemic by year 2030 per *WHO*. What can you do about that? Believe in God—boldly step up to the task you must do to liberate yourself and others from addictive habits from foods, drinks and doubts.

Its finally your turn to discover how you can lose weight using NAPS. Embracing LUCK. Learning in the "30-day Lose Weight Plan". You will lose the weights. If you still have more weight to lose at the end of the initial 30 days, now that you know what to do, continue the process until you reach your 'big' desired weight or BMI. Slim, fit and sassy and congratulations!

In writing this book, I did a survey to address the concerns of people. **There are 30 Survey questions answered in this book** that were asked about how to lose weight using, Natural Appetite-control Products and Supplements-NAPS. How to use the products ecetra.

There are eleven Natural Appetite-control Products and Supplements - NAPS to Lose Weight Everyday, outlined in this Book. This was the primary focus of this book. See the Introduction Section for the products and supplements outlined.

LIVE-LIFE UNDER CHRIST KNOWLEDGE. Acronymed LUCK. This is the secondary focus of this book. In this book, you are encouraged to do the following:-

1. **EMBRACE LUCK TO SUCCEED IN LIFE.**

   You will see the word LUCK mentioned throughout this book and especially during the "30-Day Lose Weight Everyday Plan".

2. **USE NAPS DAILY TO LOSE WEIGHT.**

3. **START THE "30-DAY LOSE WEIGHT EVERYDAY PLAN"**

   It is designed to daily give you support and encouragment to help inspire you to stay on track until you achieve your desired weight loss goals.

   30 encouraging Bible text and 30 motivational and uplifting written guides. These will come via your email each day to help you become a weight loss winner. If you do not need this, don't be mad. Be glad for those who asked for it and need it.

USING THE NATURAL APPETITE-CONTROL PRODUCTS AND SUPPLEMENTS

NAPS requires no special recipes. One scoop of the TrimShake, has the nutrients of a meal, therefore, do not overuse. These products are easy to use. Just follow the printed directions on the package.

For the TrimShakes, just simply add liquids which could be water, milk or your favorite yogurt. You can also blend in your favorite fruits and even vegetables. There is an example in the Proper Diet Bonus Section in this book.

The **Slim & Sassy Chewing Gum** can be used anytime; between meals or as you desire.

Isn't it just an awesome feeling to know that even before the day we were born, our God, already had a plan for our success in health, wealth, worship splendor and every thing else we need? Our question, "How to be Heathy Everyday", was answered by the God of heaven from creation week when he created healthy plants, fruits, vegetables, nuts, water, air, sunlight, the support systems we would need and everything else.

We all have unique responsibilities in supporting and maintaining our bodies. Use the information in this book and on the corresponding website to lose weight and keep it off for life. Embrace the wellness lifestyle, use NAPS because they naturally support a lifetime of looking, feeling and living younger, longer.

If you doubt God's plan for your life and to help you obtain that life, come with me on a journey. Don't be foolish like I was by delaying your assignment. Jumpstart it right now. Here's a true reminder that God asked me to tell you. Its in, Isaiah 41: 13 *"For I, the Lord your God, will hold your right hand, saying to you, 'Fear not, I will help you.".*

You are here to succeed to lose weight. You cannot fail when you move out of the way and allow God to lead you into your promised victories. You will also have beautiful relationships. You will have financial wealth. You will have abundant health and happiness. Take the Godly challenge and jumpstart your future with God at the center! Do it now.

Natural Appetite-control Products & Supplements - NAPS to Lose Weight Everyday

Do you need to lose five to 500 pounds? You can use these natural appetite-control products and supplements – NAPS, along with the other remedies in this Book, to "Lose Weight Everyday". The more weight you must lose, the more time it will take. Therefore, you must put more effort into losing weight. If you are willing to finally do something, God is able and has several plans for your life. There are eleven different top-rated natural products and supplements to lose weight. Thousands of people are using them everyday with amazing results. It is finally your turn. Embrace NAPS! Go to sleep. Wake up slim, fit and sassy.

QUESTION: HOW TO GET THE LOWEST PRICE?

ANSWER: NEVER PAY RETAIL PRICE FOR THE NAPS SUPPLEMENTS.

You will not have to pay retail price at this company because they have a lower price for members. Instead, get their one year Membership, cost: $35.00. Membership gets you 25% off every item you purchase for one full year. Imagine this example: Say you buy the NAPS Weight Loss Kit; Retail price $265.33. With your membership, it would be an instant savings of $66.25. The kit would cost only $199.08. You would have paid for the membership of $35 and still have money left over. You could use some of that savings to buy the Slim & Sassy Blend Chewing Gum to help curb your cravings. See the 30 Survey Question to see more about the benefits of Membership.

HOW TO START A HOME BUSINESS USING NAPS

Membership allows you to share the products with other people and get paid by the company. That is how most people start their home business using these NAPS.

Everyone I asked wants to LOOK, FEEL, LIVE YOUNGER, LONGER and have enough money to enjoy life. Unfortunately, many are too sick: mentally, physically, spiritually, nutritionally, emotionally and even financially to enjoy life. Here is an opportunity to cut your healthcare bills and replace the synthetic pills by using CPTG essential oils to support your body. CPTG oils are natural products to support and maintain the body.

IF YOU ARE SICK OR TAKING MEDICATIONS, <u>DO NOT STOP TAKING YOUR MEDICINES</u>. LET YOUR DOCTOR KNOW YOU ARE TAKING NAPS FOR HEALTH. MONITOR YOUR RESULTS. WRITE IT DOWN AND DISCUSS WITH YOUR DOCTOR. THESE PRODUCTS DO NOT HEAL, TREAT, DIAGNOSE, OR PREVENT ILLNESS.
"Lose Weight Everyday" is the goal of every overweight or obese person. There are eleven (11) proven products in our weight management program to help you manage overweight and obesity. Start now and you too could become slim, fit, and sassy.

It is possible to lose weight. Make the necessary changes in lifestyle to prevent, or even reverse some lifestyle diseases and unhealthy complications of overweight or obesity. Some individuals even decided to change from eating a lot of meats. Some stopped smoking and some started regular exercises. Some individuals may not have lifestyle diseases. Fortunately for them, they make the changes necessary to improve their health—because it is not just simply the absence of disease, but complete wellness.

"The whole philosophy of achieving happiness through great health involves much more than diet but involves what affects the mind, what foods we put in our bodies; activities of my heart, spirit, and my money. All these play a vital role in realizing best health. Think of your best health achieved as your best saving bank account. You only have in your account what you have deposited plus the interest earned. Don't worry about how to lose weight to be healthy—instead, daily work to reverse or prevent lifestyle diseases by taking better care of yourself, eating foods naturally grown, and exercising.

This is where the information in this book comes in handy for you. Rather than just receiving information on proper diet, exercise, planning, and activity, each participant is given tools such as: The "30-day Lose Weight Plan", "LUCK", NAPS, and more to help with becoming resilient, managing stress, building up but strengthening relationships, finding meaning with purpose in life, and maintaining positive change to lose weight.

There are eleven different Natural Appetite-control Products & Supplements -NAPS that are not simply short term interventions. It's an educational program designed to guide participants through the challenges associated with adopting a new lifestyle. One that's full of behaviors that bring us toward wellness, wealth and worship splendor.

Lose Weight Everyday is geared to achieve your optimal health through changing lifestyle and getting the most out of life naturally. Learning about actively working to live the best "Life Under Christ knowledge—LUCK" and enjoying all the good things of this life.

DON'T TAKE MY WORD FOR IT, READ THE RESULTS OF OTHERS IF THEY CAN DO IT, SURELY, YOU CAN TOO. JUST TRY NAPS TODAY!

WEIGHT LOSS RESULTS USING NAPS SUPPLEMENTS

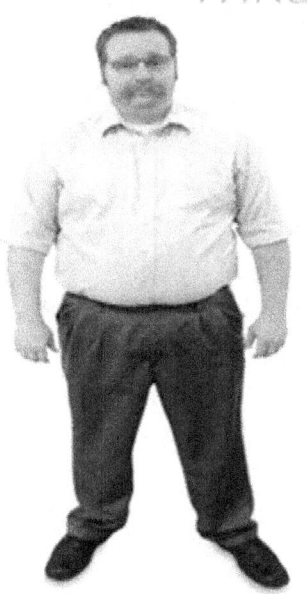
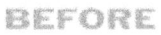
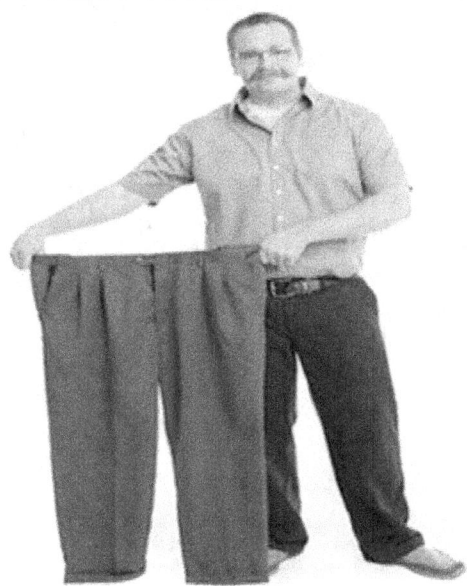

LOST **35** POUNDS IN THREE MONTHS!

BEFORE   AFTER

Ruth Rhodes

Total Weight Lost: **42** lbs.
Inches Lost: 29 inches

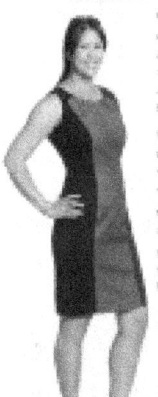

What motivated you to participate in the Slim & Sassy contest?

After having your baby, I was having a hard time with my weight. My body was not the same as before. I'd have sugar and carb cravings and was trying to work through things as a single mom.

I kept eating and the pounds kept rising and I was 100 pounds over what I had been. I was craving food & eating constantly, and I just couldn't figure out how to get myself under control.

What were some of your biggest challenges?

One of the biggest challenges I found was getting fit for good. I have two kids and no one to look out for me while I exercised.

How She Did It

Ruth kept herself supplemented with Thin-Shake and her first solution. She would then take 15-30 Slim & Sassy drops before breakfast and dinner to help curb her appetite allowing her to eat smaller portions while feeling satisfied. In spite of the recent discovery, she's been another thumbsie.

"Just keep doing it..."

Dr. Jonathan Caldwell

Total Weight Lost: **49** lbs.
Inches Lost: 27.5 inches

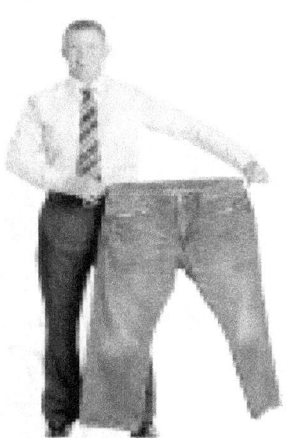

What motivated you to participate in the Slim & Sassy contest?

What was your goal during the contest?

Tips for Success

- Find a good reason to lose weight.
- Do it for your lifestyle change.
- Exercise every day even if it's only for a few minutes.

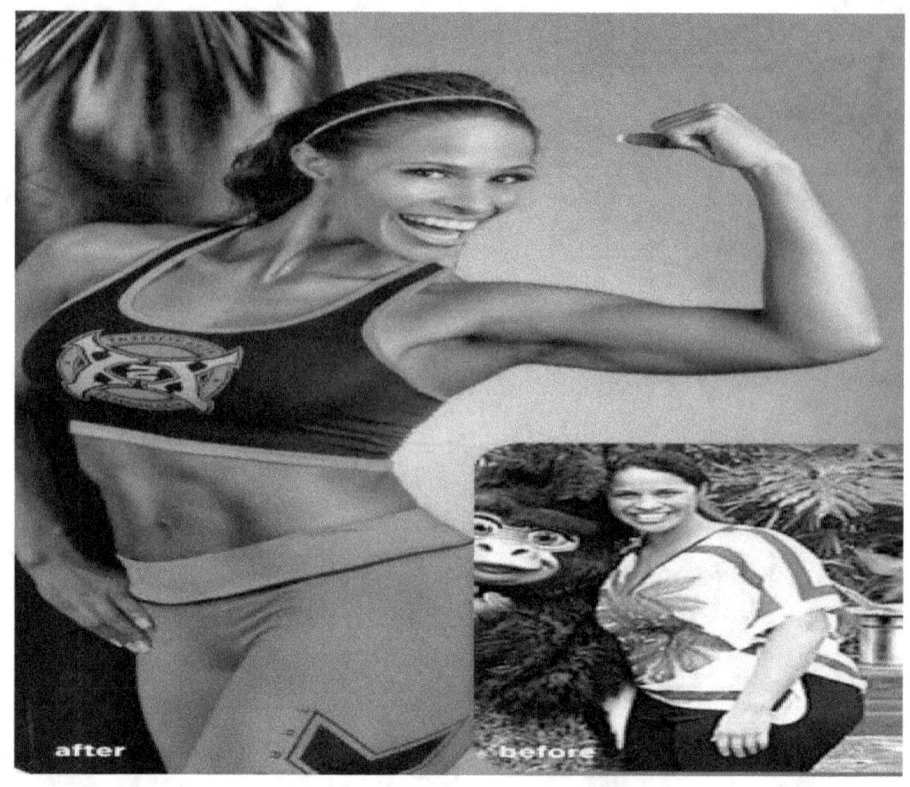

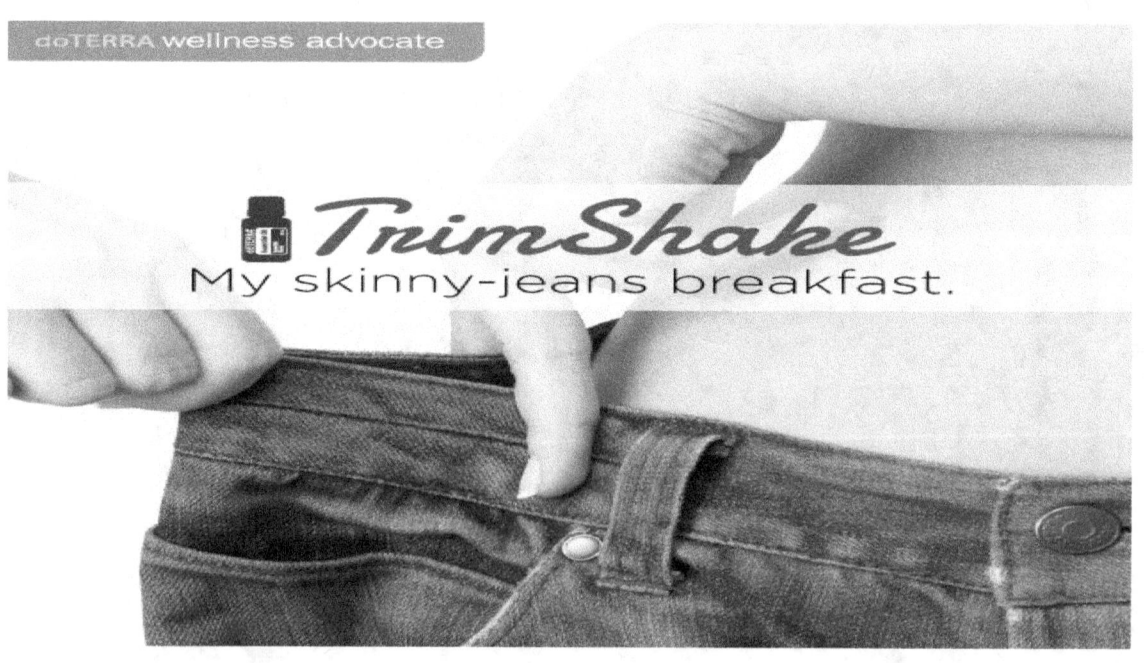

Wes Hobson (How to increase energy for professional athletes)

During his 12-year career as a professional triathlete, Wes Hobson garnered 35 first-place finishes, 60 top-three finishes, and 96 top-five finishes. He was also the first American to win a World Cup Triathlon. Overall, he has competed in 220 races. He retired from the sport of triathlon in 2001, and coached high-level triathletes for 6 ears. Currently, Wes stays fit with a variety of exercise regiments and uses a multitude of dōTERRA products to maintain his health.

Kyle Kirschbaum (How to have a great weight loss)

An entrepreneur and father of five young boys, Kyle Kirschbaum started his fitness journey when one of his businesses failed in 2010. He realized that during difficult times, he couldn't control a lot of aspects of life, but he could be in control of his nutrition and fitness. So, he went to work. Today, Kyle is passionate about sharing his journey with other fathers, husbands, and entrepreneurs who want to be in the best shape possible, but need help getting started and learning how to fit their fitness routines around their families and businesses. See which of the NAPS products he uses.

Dana Moore (Video on What? Why? How? To Lose Weight using NAPS)

Dana Moore is a wellness enthusiast and busy mom of four. She has mastered the art of incorporating healthy habits into her existing routine and approaches her wellness goals with practicality. She attributes her abilities to a BA in education and her certification as a healing foods specialist. You can frequently find Dana preparing healthy snacks and meals, working out, and teaching others how to do the same.

Jessica Moultrie (Video on Kids Nutrition)

Jessica Moultrie is a lifelong athlete, health and fitness connoisseur, and dōTERRA Wellness Advocate. A Division I college athlete, Jessica played soccer for the University of South Carolina. She is now an enthusiastic CrossFitter. In addition to her own fitness regimen, Jessica works hard to make sure her children are healthy and happy athletes. Her daughter Olivia is the first girl ever to train with the boys at the US Soccer Development Academy.

Ange Peters (Great Video how to do the math to lose weight naturally)

Ange Peters is a holistic health coach and dōTERRA Wellness Advocate who has spent much of her life learning about fitness, nutrition, and wellness. Ange is also a certified personal trainer and natural nutritionist. She tries to approach every aspect of life in a healthy way. In addition to living her life as healthy and happily as possible, Ange is passionate about educating people to become their own health advocates.

Dr. Damian Rodriguez, DHSc, MS

Dr. Damian Rodriguez holds a doctorate in Health Sciences from A.T. Still University, where he focused his research on obesity. He also holds a B.S. in Nutritional Science, a Master of Science in Exercise Physiology with an emphasis in athletic performance, as well as numerous professional certifications in exercise and nutrition.

Prior to joining dōTERRA, he worked in public health and as a strength coach and nutritionist for professional and collegiate athletes. Dr. Rodriguez has also served as a mentor to autistic teens, having lived with Asperger's syndrome himself—an autism spectrum disorder. He is a lifelong athlete who has competed in everything from powerlifting to triathlons and is passionate about helping others achieve total wellness." *Source: dōTERRA*

INTRODUCTION

ELEVEN NATURAL REMEDIES TO LOSE WEIGHT EVERYDAY
30 Survey Questions Answered About NAPS

"Weight management is one of the most critical factors in physical, emotional, and psychological well-being. Whether you want to lose a few pounds for the upcoming beach season or more for long-term health, the fundamentals of weight management are the same. Focusing on proper nutrition and supporting your body's inherent metabolic processes, dōTERRA has developed a system to ensure that your weight loss plan is healthy and easy to maintain. *

Maintaining a healthy weight is a side effect of a philosophy focused on positive lifestyle choices. There are myriad of reasons why an individual has too much fat. You eat too much, you exercise too little, you are under too much stress, or you are under a toxic load. A little knowledge, some dedication, and a few innovative products to help along the way, and weight management is a very attainable goal.

dōTERRA's weight management program is unique in that it is not an extreme diet or exercise program, but a step toward a lifestyle that will ensure sustainable change. Lifestyle changes following the healthy lifestyle pyramid, plus a little boost from Slim & Sassy® products, is the convenient and effective way to manage your weight, naturally and long term. *" *Contributed by Damian Rodriguez, DHSc, MS*

----

†Appethyl is a registered trademark of Greanleaf Medical AB; EssentraTrim is a registered trademark of NutraGenesis LLC; and Solathin is a registered trademark of Cyvex Nutrition. All other words with a trademark or registered trademark symbol are trademarks or registered trademarks of dōTERRA Holdings, LLC.

Who Else Wants to be Slim, Fit and Sassy?

Based on the norm in our present society, all hands should be going up. Here's the sad reality of the day, presently, obesity is fast becoming the new normal and the second leading cause of death in America. Let us be the ones who kill obesity first before it kills us. Nobody else can help us completely but ourselves through Christ who is our only help. We must have His Holy Sprit who empowers us to take the necessary actions needed to stop overweight and obesity because obesity kills!

I used to be overweight a few years ago until my clothes couldn't fit me well anymore. As a nurse, I felt unworthy to educate other people about achieving great health when I looked like someone who was overweight. I felt like a big hypocrite and that led me to change a lot of things about my lifestyle.

I wanted to walk for a few minutes without feeling so tired and out of breath. Is it really because of my physical condition, particularly my body weight and figure? In nursing school, I remembered how sad It was for me to see that my slim friends could run up the subway stairs while I struggled. I was getting too fat and something had to be done about that. I told myself, I was becoming unhappy and unhealthy and excuses had to stop.

I wanted to feel happy, healthy, and satisfied. I made an effort to lose weight and get rid of excess fats. Thankfully, with an ounce of willingness, a cup of patience, and a spoonful of determination, I lost weight? When people said to me, "tell me your secret," that was like special music to my ears. Plus in the nursing profession, I wanted to be an example to patients. I practiced what I preached. I ate what I knew improved health.

I have traveled the path of overweight and unhappiness in a single journey; it wasn't really a smooth ride – a trip not worth remembering. But, on the other hand, without that experience, I wouldn't have been in my position now – happy and contented with my weight. I used this overweight setback as a setup for great health comback. And now I am here to encourage you dear overweight or obese reader, that your change starts the moment you say: that's enough. The moment you say, I can and I will change and start to do something about it!

Thus, if I can do it, so can you. I don't want anyone else to feel what I felt before – unhappy, unhealthy, and insecure. Or worse, might even suffer from complications and other illnesses. Being fat, overweight, or obese is unhealthy, both in the mind, in the body, in the pockets and the spirit. We know it. we've been there, right?

Now, come with me on a 30-day journey where we can change not only our body size, weight, and figure, but our lives as well. There's nothing more wonderful than being able to do what you want to do or to go where you'd like to go without feeling sick. That is real happiness and contentment. And like me, you too can achieve weight loss naturally. The best prize will be that, you can find nice clothes in any store without having to make do with 'baggy' clothes that is so large, it makes you look unwell.

YOU MAY ASK ME, WHY THIS 'LOSE WEIGHT EVERYDAY BOOK'?

I will answer you honestly by giving you the facts—only the facts.

You Need to Know the Skinny on Your Fat

Before you can get started losing fat, you need to understand what body fat is and where it comes from. Your body's preferred sources of energy are dietary carbohydrates, fats, and proteins. However, when you consume more than you use, those calories are stored in fat cells for later use.

Fat cells are formed by converting tissue stem cells into adipocytes that swell up like balloons with dietary lipids. When caloric needs exceed available free calories from the food we eat, calories stored as lipids in fat cells are released into the blood stream for energy. Managing a healthy body fat percentage includes slowing down the production of new fat cells and increasing the burn rate of calories stored in body fat.

The only solution to lose weight everyday is to store fewer calories as fat by following these three equations:

Eat Less + Exercise More = Lean Body Mass

Calories In -→ Fat Stored -→

Calories Out -→ Fat Released

SUMMARY

The body absorbs the oils the fastest breathing (inhalation). The second fastest way is through rubbing the oils on the bottom of feet or on the ears.

The life expectancy of a cell is about 120 days or as I tell -people, 4 months. If the cell walls get thickened, oxygen cannot get through to nourish the cell. Cells also divide, making duplicate cells.

What will happen if the dividing cell is diseased? The duplicated cells will be diseased as well. The important thing here is to stop the mutation of the diseased cell by feeding the body with healthy nutrients. The NAPS essential oils products have the ability to penetrate the cell membrane thus carrying nutrients into the cell to improve the health of the cell.

Losing weight and keeping it off requires a lifestyle change and not returning to the old habits. Begin by asking yourself what triggers your bad eating habits?

1. Is it the fast foods eaten everyday for breakfast, lunch, even dinner and snacks?
2. Is it the candy or snacks that is my weakness?
3. By skipping meals and letting myself get too hungry, when its meal time, I eat too much?
4. Do I buy too much unhealthy foods so, when I want to eat, I have no healthy choices?
5. Do I just let my body go as if "who cares if I'm fat and getting sick from it"?

Whatever your reason to be overweight or obese. Write it down and confront it right now.

YOUR 30 SURVEY QUESTIONS ANSWERED HERE

1. WHY LOSE WEIGHT?

In a world where slim, fit and sassy, were once the expected standard of society; overweight and obesity are now the new normal. So, let's go lose weight everyday usisng affordable NAPS, and secure LUCK! Check out my website, http://lose-weight-everyday.com/ to get the facts to lose weight anyday.

2. IS THIS ANOTHER DIET PLAN?

No, not a diet plan but Natural Appetite-control Products and Supplements - NAPS!

So, in April 2008, some honest people who believed in doing right in the sight of God and bringing pure unadulterated CPTG Certified Pure Therapeutic Grade® Essentials Oils to the world began a company and conducted their "Business Under God" acronymed BUG.

Today those people have created one of the biggest essential oils companies in the world. They are the industry's leaders in providing the entire world with CPTG oils. They go all over the world and 'bug' (track) the best trees. Teaching the natives how to grow these trees correctly to get the very best essential oils. Read more about this company in the Introduction Section.

3.   WHAT ARE NAPS?

Natural Appetite-control Products & Supplements (NAPS) helps manage appetite and uplifts mood. Supports healthy metabolism of fat and energy production. Supports healthy insulin response and management of toxins. Helps the body deflate current fat cells and stops the body from producing more fat cells

Some of the products--TrimShake has Sensoril that helps control cortisol levels which triggers accumulation of fat around stomach, hips and thighs. It also helps reduce stress-induced appetite, carbohydrate cravings and supports cellular energy production.

There are eleven weight management products that our company offers and each one is explained in the Introduction section of this book. Here is a list of the weight management products.

1. Slim & Sassy® Liquid
2. Slim & Sassy® Softgels
3. Slim & Sassy® Metabolic Gum
4a Slim & Sassy® TrimShake—Chocolate
4b Slim & Sassy® TrimShake—Orange Cream
4c Slim & Sassy® TrimShake—Vanilla
5. Slim & Sassy® V Shake
6. Slim & Sassy® New You Kit
7. Slim & Sassy® Trim Kit - 1 Chocolate, 1 Vanilla
8. Slim & Sassy® Trim Kit - 2 Chocolate Trim Shakes
9. Slim & Sassy® Trim Kit - 2 Vanilla Trim Shakes
10. Slim & Sassy® Trim Kit—2 V Shake
11. Lifelong Vitality Complex

4.   WHAT ARE THE NAPS PRODUCTS MADE OF?

✓ Natural Appetite-control Products & Supplements—NAPS are made from CPTG Certified Pure Therapeutic Grade® Essential Oils plus natural products such as fruits and vegetables. I know that's a mouth full but come follow me as I break it down for you. To work with committed partners and to ensure the best growing conditions, dōTERRA sources essential oils from across the globe. With an ever-expanding product line that includes over 100 different essential oils sourced from over 40 nations, dōTERRA truly offers Earth's best gifts.

5.   WHAT ARE ESSENTIAL OILS?

Essential oils are natural aromatic compounds found in the seeds, bark, stems, roots, and flowers of plants. They can be both beautifully and powerfully fragrant, eliciting profound emotional responses. Yet the use of essential oils goes well beyond their fragrant appeal. Used throughout history for their medicinal and therapeutic benefits, essential oils can be used as natural alternatives in holistic self-care practices. Their unique chemistry allows them to be used aromatically and applied topically to the skin, while other essential oils can be used as dietary aids to promote vitality and well-being.

(Meaning "Gift of the Earth") essential oils represent the safest, purest essential oils available in the world today. Each of dōTERRA's CPTG Certified Pure Therapeutic Grade® essentials oils are carefully extracted by a global network of skilled growers, distillers, and chemists ensuring a consistently powerful user experience. They are 100% pure aromatic extracts and contain no artificial ingredients and are tested to be free of contaminants such as pesticides or other chemical residues.

We welcome your participation in our mission to share the life-enhancing benefits of therapeutic-grade essential oils with the world. Your path to a new philosophy of wellness begins by opening a bottle.

6.   WHERE ARE THE NAPS PRODUCTS MADE?

The dōTERRA Difference

Start with the growers. While others in the essential oil industry cut corners during the planting, growing, and harvesting process, or even try to "extend" pure oils by adding less expensive ingredients, dōTERRA is uncompromisingly selective.

While the temptation for a company as large as dōTERRA may be to buy large plots of land and mass produce oils, dōTERRA places great value on the expert knowledge of local farmers—many of whom have nurtured essential oil plants for generations. dōTERRA recruits their experts from a Global Botanical Network and, in so doing, supports thousands of jobs around the world.

Through dōTERRA's Global Botanical Network of farmers and essential oil producers, dōTERRA has leveraged the experience of skilled partners around the world to create the optimal supply chain for production, distillation, and distribution, enabling dōTERRA to supply these essential oils directly to you and your loved ones.

Finally, the proper natural appetite-control products and supplements manufactured in Utah, America by the one and only dōTERRA.

---

7. ARE THEY 100% ORGANIC NEVER PROCESSED?

You and your family deserve only the most pure, potent, and effective oils on earth. dōTERRA takes great pride in sourcing them to you. NAPS Essential oils products represent the safest, purest essential oils available in the world today.

CPTG Certified Pure Therapeutic Grade® essentials oils are carefully extracted by a global network of skilled growers, distillers, and chemists ensuring a consistently powerful user experience. They are 100% pure aromatic extracts and contain no artificial ingredients and are tested to be free of contaminants such as pesticides or other chemical residues.

dōTERRA's state-of-the-art lab uses the most advanced testing methods to verify the purity and potency of its essential oils. After the aromatic compounds are distilled from the plant material, each batch is scrupulously tested to ensure that it meets CPTG Certified Pure Therapeutic Grade® standards.

dōTERRA developed this rigorous criterion to certify that its oils contain no added fillers, synthetic ingredients, or harmful contaminants. Utilizing its own facilities, as well as trusted third-party labs, dōTERRA essential oils undergo the CPTG process to ensure that customers receive the highest quality oil, every time.

---

8. HOW DO I KNOW THE PRODUCTS ARE SAFE TO USE?

THE MOST TESTED, BECOMES THE MOST TRUSTED.

The dōTERRA mission hinges on discovering and developing the world's

highest quality essential oils, and we stay at the forefront of scientific advances by partnering with selected academic, industry, and scientific institutions.

Each batch of essential oils goes through a battery of rigorous and definitive tests. These tests include the following:

Gas Chromatography and Mass Spectroscopy (GC/MS) have been touted as the standard for essential oil testing, and while they remain an early indicator of quality, they are not a definitive indicator of quality.

Organoleptic Assessments: In this phase, essential oil chemists, manufacturing engineers, and quality technicians manually assess the appearance, aroma, and color of each essential oil.

Specific Gravity: The specific gravity portion of the testing process compares the volume-to-weight ratio to reference standards to verify oil quality and purity.

Gas Chromatography/ Mass Spectroscopy (GC/MS): During this stage, molecules are separated and identified to ensure that the chemistry of the oil matches the expected chemical profile.

Fourier Transform Infrared Spectroscopy (FTIR): FTIR testing uses infrared light to analyze the material composition of an oil to determine if it meets dōTERRA's established standards.

Optical Rotation: Optical rotation then tests for chirality (the orientation of molecules), using instrumentation to twist essential oil molecules to identify synthetic additives that GC/MS testing would not detect.

Refractive Index: A refractometer is used to determine the essential oil's refractive index—a measurement of how light spreads through a specific substance—to ensure the essential oil meets dōTERRA's established standards.

Contamination Testing: Batches that meet the physical testing criteria are then run through a series of on-site contamination tests by expert microbiologists to confirm that there are no harmful contaminants. The oils are tested for potentially harmful microorganisms, heavy metals, and pesticides to certify safe use when proper usage guidelines are followed.

Stability Testing: dōTERRA also conducts on-going stability testing to ensure that essential oils will maintain their purity and efficacy for the length of their intended use. In this series of tests, chambers that alter temperature and humidity are used to analyze how essential oils react when exposed to different atmospheric conditions for extended periods of time. This testing protocol ensures that dōTERRA essential oils will continue to provide safe and effective benefits for years

We welcome your participation in our mission to share the life-enhancing benefits of therapeutic-grade essential oils with the world. Your path to a new philosophy of wellness begins by opening these products.

9.   HOW TO USE THE NAPS PRODUCTS

NAPS Essential Oils have unique chemistry allowing them to be used in three ways.

1. **Aromatically**: inhale or use a diffuser.
2. **Topically** to the skin, massage, under the feet, immune system support;
3. **Internally** as dietary aids to promote vitality, well-being and weight loss.

If the essential oils get into the eyes by accident or if they burn the skin a little, do not attempt to use water to wash off. Oil and water does not mix. The water will drive the oil deeper into the skin. Always dilute with oil such as vegetable oil or fractionated coconut oil.

Remember the CPTG oils are pure, use with caution until you know how you respond to them. Less is better, so use one to three drops in your liquid. Topically, dilute with vegetable oils and no more than six drops at a time. Mix and rub in clockwise direction

10.   HOW DO CPTG ESSENTIAL OILS WORK?
Contains a superfood blend that helps support overall health and wellness

 Smell the Aroma 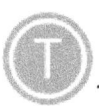 Topical Uses   Take Internally 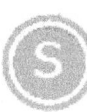 Sensitive

11.   WHO NEEDS NAPS PRODUCTS—ESSENTIAL OILS?
If you are overweight or obese, sick with lifestyle diseases or taking multiple medications but cannot get rid of your obesity, then you need NAPS.

Do you find yourself asking questions such as the ones below?

- Why do I have to take all these synthetic drugs everyday? What can I do to lose the weight and feel better?
- Why am I always sick, tired, feeble, weak, energy-less and broke?
- Is my life always going to be this difficult?
- Why can't I have great relationships, or have confidence, or be calm?

- Why can't I seem to get ahead and stay ahead?
- Why do I work so hard, and yet have so little to show for it? I want a change...BUT I am so fat and hurting all the time.
- What must I do to lose weight, be happy and fell healthy?

Many of these obese individuals struggling to find the proper products that could help them curb the appetite, reduce the cravings and lose weight will be glad to have NAPS. Finally, the proven natural products to lose weight fast and keep it off for life when you use them as directed.

NAPS made from CPTG oils are 50 – 70 times more powerful than herbs and therefore, inhibit the growth of bacteria and viruses in cells. These products inhibit your cravings for sugar, high carbs, salt, fatty foods that led you down the obesity pathway. NAPS are very effective. They are safe to use,100% pure. Give NAPS a try today!

12. WHAT ARE THE STANDARD OF SAFETY & STRINGENCY?

The standard of safety is equally stringent and efficacy are applied to all the essential wellness products. Guided by our Scientific Advisory Board, and this company uses only top development and manufacturing partners who maintain GMP certification and enjoy industry reputation for quality and superior innovation. Each essential oil or oil product is certain to surpass customer satisfaction and performance expectations.

Scientific Experts and Advisors

Along with an impressive staff that oversees the day-to-day testing and chemical processes for dōTERRA essential oils, dōTERRA has assembled the industry's most distinguished group of advisors.

Our unrivaled scientific experts and advisors include the world's foremost authorities in essential oil chemistry, botany, microbiology, physiology, research science, nutritional science, and nutraceuticals.

Learn more about our Scientific Experts and Advisors

At the 2015 annual convention, Dr. David Hill announced that there were 16 top scientists working on testing of essential oils and developing more products to support the body and maintain it. The science behind the CPTG Certified Pure Therapeutic Grade essential oils.

Join dōTERRA executives and Wellness Advocate leaders as they share how to live an active healthy lifestyle through proper nutrition, exercise, stress management in partnership with informed self-care and proactive medical care. Be educated on how to use essential oils and supplements to care for your family in a safe and effective way. Special new product offers will be available to event attendees only, this will be an event you won't want to miss!

Medical Advisory Board

dōTERRA has assembled a medical advisory board of top experts in fields ranging from dentistry to orthopedic surgery. dōTERRA works directly with these healthcare professionals and the larger medical community in developing and advancing the uses of essential oils in clinical environments.

13. TELL US ABOUT THE COMPANY?

dōTERRA International, LLC produces and distributes exceptionally high quality CPTG Certified Pure Therapeutic Grade essential oils through more than three million independent distributors, also known as Wellness Advocates, around the world. In addition to a premium line of essential oils used by individuals and health-care professionals alike, the company also offers products that are naturally safe, purely effective, and infused with CPTG essential oils, including personal care and spa products, nutritional supplements, and healthy living products.

Growth Milestones May 2008 – dōTERRA founded December 2008 – dōTERRA reaches $1 million in sales 2009 – dōTERRA has first $1 million month

2012 – dōTERRA has regular $1 million days March 2013 – dōTERRA breaks ground on state-of-the-art corporate headquarters July 2014 – dōTERRA celebrates 1,000,000 Wellness Advocates.

August 2014 – dōTERRA corporate headquarters Phase 1 completed June 2015 – Phase 2 of the corporate headquarters is complete bringing 383,000 total square feet of professional office and manufacturing space online 2015 – dōTERRA establishes Esseterre Bulgaria EOOD, a farming and distilling operation in eastern Bulgaria 2015 – dōTERRA reaches more than $1 billion in sales June 2016 - dōTERRA celebrates 3,000,000 Wellness Advocates August 2016 –

dōTERRA ships products to customers in nearly 100 countries and has corporate offices in 17 countries. Leading the Industry in retention.

dōTERRA enjoys a 68 percent retention rate, compared to a direct selling industry average near 10 percent. Why?
1. Customers and Wellness Advocates are satisfied with product value
2. High satisfaction levels lead to a desire to share products and success with others
3. Product sales leaders recognize the value of dōTERRA's powerful compensation plan

People and Places

dōTERRA completed a new global headquarters in Pleasant Grove, Utah, USA in 2015. dōTERRA employs more than 1850 people in day-to-day corporate operations. More than 1600 of these employees work from the new campus in support of the more than three million independent distributors around the world.

14. WHAT ARE THE COMPANY INNOVATIVE STANDARDS?

An Innovative Standards

dōTERRA CPTG Certified Pure Therapeutic Grade essential oils represent the safest and most beneficial oils available in the world today. For an oil to be CPTG Certified Pure Therapeutic Grade the oil must be: Pure and natural, with aromatic compounds carefully extracted from plants Free from fillers or artificial ingredients; no dilution of active qualities Free of contaminants, pesticides, or chemical residues.

Rigorously tested for standards of chemical composition Cross tested using mass spectrometry and gas chromatography to ensure exact purity and composition potency Sourced by a global network of leading essential oil chemists and growers to ensure correct species, growth in ideal environments, and that raw plant materials were carefully harvested at the right time

dōTERRA Co-Impact Sourcing dōTERRA works to improve lives and communities throughout the world. Many of the essential oils offered by dōTERRA are sourced in developing countries, where the growers and distillers are often at the mercy of third parties.

dōTERRA Co-Impact Sourcing helps create coalitions of growers and distillers that ensure local communities receive fair and timely payments to support their families and communities. dōTERRA works with these coalitions to provide the resources, tools, and training necessary to ensure a long-lasting partnership.

dōTERRA focuses philanthropic efforts through the dōTERRA Healing Hands Foundation. Its mission is to bring healing and hope to the world, for lives free of disease and poverty, and ultimately to teach impoverished cultures to be self-reliant.

The foundation is supported by contributions from dōTERRA independent distributors known as Wellness Advocates, retail and preferred customers, company employees and executives, and others who share our vision. Donations are collected through monthly contributions, onetime contributions, and select product sales. For more information visit Healing Hands.

The Healing Hands Foundation has been involved in many projects, including the following: Micro-credit loans providing renewable funding for entrepreneurs in developing communities. Clean water wells and programs. Building and revitalizing schools and clinics. Medical equipment and resources for hospitals and clinics. Education on hygiene and health.

15.   What can I use to resist those mid-day munchies?

Thousands of overweight individuals are using Slim & Sassy Metabolic Blend which is designed to help manage appetite between meals.

16.   What Is the lowest price for these products

You can buy these weight loss products at the retail price but don't. Instead get a membership cost: $35.00 good for one year! Because membership gets you 25% off every item you purchase. Example: Today, say you buy a product; Retail $265.33 with the membership it would be only $199.00. Instant savings of $66.33. You would have paid for the membership and still have money left over to buy the control snack bars to eat between the meals or chewing gum or the supplement to add to your water, juice or milk throughout the day. Membership is wise shopping.

You can get a free membership value $35.00 when you purchase any of the kits. So, get one of the complete weight loss kit today and discover the privileges of membership. The savings add up fast. Your membership kit comes with all the instructions you will need to get started. If you need more information, contact us or the company where a friendly staff will be happy to assist you.

17. HOME BUSINESS: Can I Use NAPS Certified Products For That?

Because of the tremendous potential for the continued growth of dōTERRA, and because word of mouth or personal referral is the most common method of people learning about essential oils, dōTERRA is very committed to direct selling as the vehicle by which its CPTG Certified Pure Therapeutic Grade® essential oils are marketed. Direct selling is generally defined as the selling of goods away from a fixed retail location and includes personal involvement by someone experienced in the use of the goods being sold.

18. What Are the Earnings Potential Of NAPS?

When you purchase a dōTERRA Membership of $35.00, you will get a personalized website to make your purchases. Another benefit of this website, you can refer friends, family and others to your site to make purchases.

If you would like to sell the products in a "for profit business", you then participate in the monthly LRP Program. See below for what this program means.

The dōTERRA business opportunity is robust and growing. While the clear majority of Wellness Advocates are focused on the use of essential oils for the benefit of their family and friends, for those Wellness Advocates that desire to focus on developing a "for profit" business by working full time and achieving the leadership ranks, there is a significant earnings opportunity as noted below. Of course, each Wellness Advocate's actual earnings will depend on many factors including the time and effort they put into building their own dōTERRA business.

LRP dōTERRA Loyalty Rewards Program (LRP)
Q & A

19. What is the best way to get essential oils?

The best way to get essential oils is to sign up as a Wellness Advocate yourself. Once you sign up as a Wellness Advocate, you will be able to qualify for the Loyalty Rewards Program and the Product of the Month Club, which will help you to minimize your product expenses and maximize your product quantity.

20. What are benefits of signing up as a Wellness Advocate?

When you sign up as a Wellness Advocate, you can purchase dōTERRA products at wholesale prices (which is 25 percent below retail prices). You will also be able to participate in the Loyalty Rewards Program (LRP) and the Product of the Month Club.

21. What is the dōTERRA Loyalty Rewards Program (LRP)?

The dōTERRA Loyalty Rewards Program (LRP) is a program that provides free provides free product credits for monthly purchases ordered on the program. As a participant in the Loyalty Rewards Program, you will immediately begin to earn product credits that can be used as cash to purchase dōTERRA products.

The longer you participate, the more credits you can earn—up to 30% of your total monthly Loyalty Rewards purchases!

22. What are product points?

Product points are earned points that can be cashed in for more dōTERRA products through the Loyalty Rewards Program.

23. How do product points work?

Product points accumulate from each LRP order you place. The percentage of product points that you earn (ranging from 10 to 30 percent) depends on the type of enrollment kit you purchase when you sign up as a Wellness Advocate. Product point percentages will grow every quarter until you reach a maximum of 30 percent. Additionally, when you place your order online, you earn 100 percent of your shipping costs back as points.

24. How can I qualify for free product?

You can qualify for free product by participating in the Product of the Month Club.

25. What is the Product of the Month Club?

Each product has been assigned a value of Personal Volume (PV). When you purchase doTERRA products, your PV increases. When your PV reaches 125, dōTERRA will send you the pre-selected product of the month. The higher the PV of each of your orders, the more chances you will have to qualify for the product of the month and any other promotions that doTERRA offers throughout the year.

The product of the month can be earned only on the Loyalty Rewards Program by placing an order of 125 PV or more between the first and fifteenth of the month.

26. What does PV stand for?

PV stands for Personal Volume. Each dōTERRA product has been assigned a value of PV. When you purchase dōTERRA products, your PV increases.

27. Do You want to Know About Earnings Potential with NAPS?

Example: 2015 Opportunity / Earnings Disclosure Summary

A 2014 U.S. based research study by a reputable third party organization highlighted various aspects of the growth opportunity of dōTERRA® in the coming years. Key takeaways from this study include the following:

- 73 percent of the population looks to natural products to improve their health.51 percent of the general population has used essential oils.
- Of the general population, only 13 percent are familiar with dōTERRA essential oils.
- The most popular method to find out which natural product to use and how to use those products continues to be from the recommendation of a friend. This method is 50% more common than referring to an advertisement.

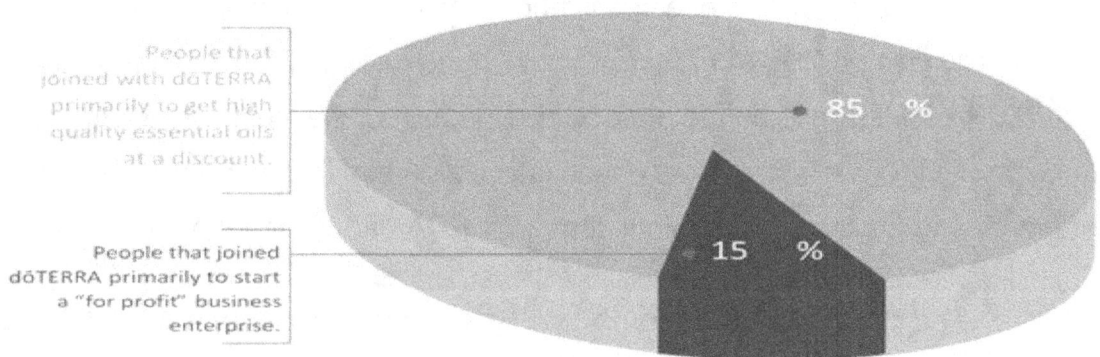

dōTERRA is an essential oils company that markets through direct selling. The above referenced study also explored dōTERRA's direct selling channel and revealed that 85 percent of the people that joined dōTERRA did so primarily to get high quality essential oils at a discount for themselves and their family. Only 15 percent joined primarily to start a "for profit" business enterprise.

Therefore, the vast majority of the approximately three million dōTERRA members around the world are primarily focused on getting access to high quality essential oils and other products offered by dōTERRA at the most reasonable price possible. dōTERRA supports this desire by having a very generous Loyalty Rewards Program that has extremely high participation rates and a near 100 percent point redemption rate by loyal consumers.

Additionally, dōTERRA offers regular promotions and other opportunities for members to purchase products at a discount. The above referenced study of dōTERRA members showed that after the quality of the company's essential oils, the next three things respondents believe the company does best include: being a values-based organization, providing great customer support, and offering a compelling compensation plan.

Supporting this extremely high focus on products, the dōTERRA compensation plan provides a robust earnings opportunity for all Wellness Advocates. Wellness Advocates are dōTERRA members that have enrolled to receive the deepest product discounts. While more than 85% of all dōTERRA members join to focus primarily on the ability to buy high quality oils at a discount, they can and do earn commissions for their efforts based on the sales of product within their organization.

During 2015, the company paid commissions to approximately 225,000 Wellness Advocates in the United States which is approx. 20% of all U.S. based dōTERRA members that made a purchase from the company during the year.

Specifically, 12% of dōTERRA members do not become Wellness Advocates and cannot earn commissions. Wellness Advocates classified by the rank of Consultant account for 74% of all dōTERRA members and don't generally enroll other members or earn commissions. Entry-level Wellness Advocates with the rank of Manager, Director and Executive earn up to $1,600 annually in commissions and account for 9% of all dōTERRA members. At the mid-level ranks of Elite and Premier (4% of all dōTERRA members), Wellness Advocates learn about participating in dōTERRA as a business and are almost always doing the business on a part-time basis. Average annual earnings for these ranks range from $3,950 to $9,950 per year.

28.   What's the Highest Levels in the Commission Plan?

The highest levels in the commission plan are the leadership ranks and the 2015 average annual earnings for these ranks are shown in the following chart. Within these ranks are some of dōTERRA members that conduct business on a full-time basis. This chart shows the rank, the average annual earnings of Wellness Advocates paid at that rank during 2015, and the percent of people within these leadership ranks who were paid at that specific rank in the United States:

Rank	Average Annual Earnings	Percent of Leaders
Silver	$26,600	62%
Gold	$59,000	23%
Platinum	$115,000	5%
Diamond	$205,000	7%
Blue Diamond	$462,000	2%
Presidential Diamond	$1,353,000	<1%

dōTERRA experienced tremendous growth during 2015 in large part due to an increase in the number of people achieving leadership ranks globally

Rank	Number of First Time Rank Achievement in 2015
Silver	3,096
Gold	1,020
Platinum	435
Diamond	266
Blue Diamond	60
Presidential Diamond	13

*Results not typical.

29. Are There Any Bonuses?

☐

When you purchase any kit, you get a free membership. A value of $35.00. Membership has its rewards. At dōTERRA there are several rewards to owning a membersjip.

30. What benefits will you receive by choosing to purchase an enrollment kit as your membership?

When you choose to purchase an enrollment kit as your membership, the 35 US dollar membership fee will be waived, and you will receive a substantial discount on doTERRA products.

Becoming a dōTERRA Wellness Advocate is an amazing opportunity to purchase CPTG essential oils at 25% below the retail cost. With an enrollment charge of $35, you will have access to many business and product tools that will help you enjoy the benefits of living, sharing, and building with dōTERRA.

When you become a Wellness Advocate, you will be given a wholesale membership number and will be prompted to create a password. Once you have obtained your membership ID number, you can purchase products online by visiting mydoterra.com or by contacting member services toll free at 800-411-8151.

Creating an Order: You have two options as a Wellness Advocate when you create your orders.

Standard Order: This type of order can be placed at any time online or through member services. A standard order is a wholesale order that qualifies you for 25% in savings.

Loyalty Rewards Order (LRP): This is the smartest way to purchase products at dōTERRA. This is an auto-ship program that not only allows you to purchase products at wholesale prices, but also allows you the opportunity to earn 10% to 30% of your total purchase in free product points.

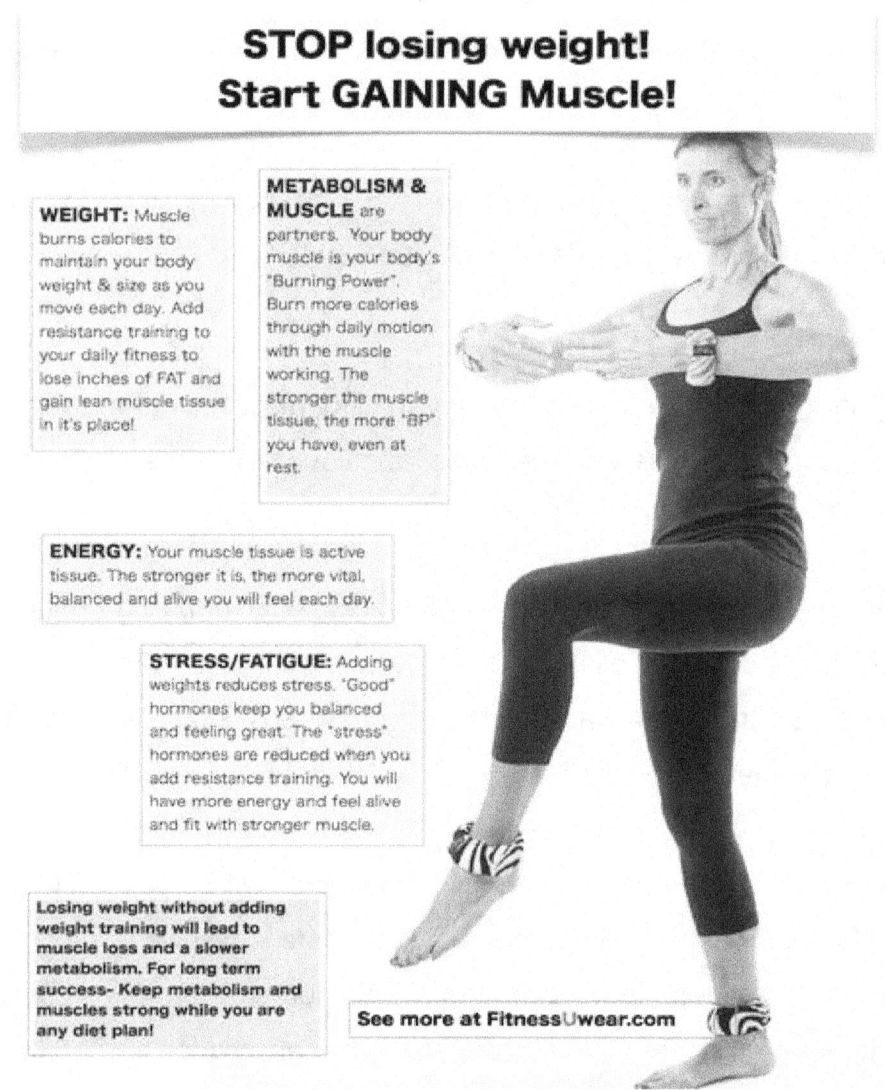

ELEVEN NATURAL PROVEN APPETITE-CONTROL PRODUCTS AND SUPPLEMENTS TO LOSE WEIGHT WITHOUT DIETING

PRODUCT 1:

Slim & Sassy® Metabolic Blend

"Slim & Sassy Metabolic Blend is your first line of defense against weight-gain, helping to naturally promote healthy metabolism. *

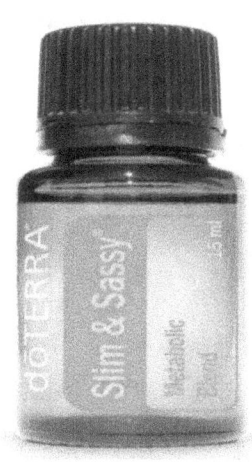

The proprietary blend of Grapefruit, Lemon, Peppermint, Ginger, and Cinnamon Bark essential oils provides a flavorful way to manage the inevitable hunger and mood variations that accompany your weight management plan. When taken internally, it helps to

Figure 1Slim & Sassy Metabolic Blend

support healthy metabolism, keeping your natural fat-burning mechanisms working at peak efficiency. A few drops in four ounces of your favorite beverage before meals or in a Slim & Sassy TrimShake as a meal or snack replacement can promote the health of your body's natural weight management mechanisms and help control urges to overeat." *Contributed by Damian Rodriguez, DHSc, MS*

Primary Benefits

- Promotes healthy metabolism*
- Helps manage hunger cravings*
- Calms your stomach and lifts your mood
- Diuretic, stimulant, and calorie free*

Ingredients: Grapefruit Peel, Lemon Peel, Peppermint Plant, Ginger Root, and Cinnamon Bark essential oils.

Aromatic Description: Warm, spicy, herbal

Designed to help boost your metabolism and manage hunger cravings, Slim & Sassy Metabolic Blend can be used as part of a weight management plan when combined with exercise and healthy eating. *

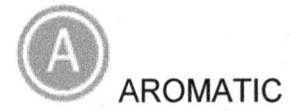 AROMATIC 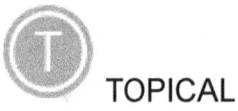 TOPICAL 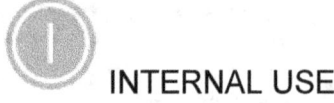 INTERNAL USE 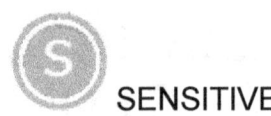 SENSITIVE

Part Number: 31370001
Size: 15 Ml   Wholesale: $24.50   Retail: $32.67   PV: 24.50

Click to Buy Now: Slim & Sassy® Metabolic Blend
or Copy and Paste in Browser: http://bit.ly/2IEZ8V5

Description

Slim & Sassy, our proprietary metabolic blend, combines powerful essential oils known to promote a healthy metabolism in a natural way. * The flavorful blend of Slim & Sassy helps manage hunger throughout the day while supporting healthy metabolism and promoting a positive mood. * Slim & Sassy contains Grapefruit, Lemon, Peppermint, Ginger, and Cinnamon. When taken with a healthy eating and exercise plan, Slim & Sassy Metabolic Blend can help you reach your weight management goals. *

Uses

- Add to water or tea and drink before working out for a revitalizing energy boost. *
- Consume before meals to help control appetite and overeating. *
- Perfect for any healthy weight management program. *
- Add a few drops to Slim & Sassy TrimShake or V Shake.

Directions for Use

Diffusion: Use three to four drops in the diffuser of your choice.
Internal use: Dilute four drops in 4 fl. oz. of liquid.
Topical use: Apply one to two drops to desired area.

Dilute with doTERRA Fractionated Coconut Oil to minimize any skin sensitivity.

Cautions

Possible skin sensitivity. Keep out of reach of children. If you are pregnant, nursing, or under a doctor's care, consult your physician. Avoid contact with eyes, inner ears, and sensitive areas. Avoid sunlight or UV rays for up to 12 hours after applying product.

Statements with asterisks refer to internal use. All others refer to aromatic or topical use.

PRODUCT 2

Slim & Sassy® Softgels

30-Days supply, take as directed on the bottle.

This is same as the metabolic blend above only that it comes in a vegetable capsule instead of in droplets.

Primary Benefits

Slim & Sassy® Softgels

- Promotes healthy metabolism*
- Helps manage hunger cravings*
- Calms your stomach and lifts your mood
- Diuretic-, stimulant-, and calorie-free*

Key Ingredients and Benefits

Grapefruit Peel: provides cleansing and detoxifying benefits*
Lemon Peel: acts as a natural cleanser and aids digestion*
Peppermint Plant: helps manage hunger cravings*
Ginger Root: may help support healthy digestion*
Cinnamon Bark: supports healthy metabolic function*

Other Ingredients

Non-GMO modified corn starch, glycerin, carrageenan, purified water, maltitol.

Slim & Sassy® Softgels

Infused with the Slim & Sassy proprietary blend, Slim & Sassy Softgels help promote a healthy metabolism and provide detoxifying benefits through an easy-to-take softgel. *Part

Number: 34270001   INTERNAL USE
Size: 90 vegetarian softgels   Wholesale: $34.50   Retail: $46.00   PV: 30

Click to Buy Now Slim & Sassy®: Metabolic Softgels
or Copy and Paste in Browser: http://bit.ly/2IEZ8V5

Description
Slim & Sassy Metabolic Blend Softgels contain dōTERRA's proprietary Slim & Sassy essential oil blend in convenient softgels to promote weight loss in a healthy, natural way. *

The flavorful blend of Slim & Sassy contains essential oils to help manage hunger throughout the day while boosting metabolism and promoting a positive mood.

Slim & Sassy contains Grapefruit and Lemon essential oils, both of which have a high limonene content to help purify and cleanse the body while Peppermint aids digestion and helps curb the appetite. *

Additionally, Ginger and Cinnamon provide healthy digestive and metabolic support. * When combined with healthy eating and exercise, Slim & Sassy Metabolic Blend can help you reach your weight management goal and maintain a healthy weight for life. * Slim & Sassy Softgels are perfect for on-the-go or for those wanting an easy and convenient way to consume Slim & Sassy essential oil blend.

Uses

Take 3 to 5 softgels throughout the day as needed.

Cautions

Keep out of reach of children. If you are pregnant, nursing, or under a doctor's care, consult your physician. Store in a cool, dry place.

*These statements have not been evaluated by the Food and Drug Administration. This product is not intended to diagnose, treat, cure, or prevent any disease.

PRODUCT 3

Slim & Sassy® Metabolic Chewing Gum

Primary Benefits

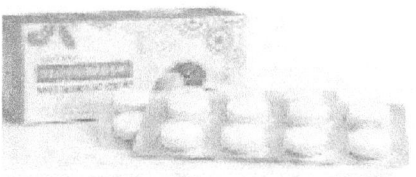

- Promotes healthy metabolism
- Helps manage hunger cravings
- Sugar free with natural sweeteners
- One drop of Slim & Sassy oil blend in every piece
- Long lasting flavor. Use between meals, reduce cravings

Figure 2 Slim & Sassy Metabolic Chewing Gum

Nutrition Facts

Amount Per Serving:
Calories 0, Total Fat 0g (0%DV), Sat. Fat 0g (0% DV), Trans Fat 0g, Cholest. 0g (0% DV), Sodium 0mg (0% DV), Total Carb. Less than 1g (0% DV), Fiber 0g (0% DV), Total Sugars

0g (0% DV), Sugar Alc. Less than 1g, Protein 0g, Vit. D (0% DV), Calcium (0% DV), Iron (0% DV), Potas. (0% DV).

Other Ingredients:

Sorbitol, Gumbase, Slim & Sassy Oil Blend (Grapefruit Peel Oil, Lemon Peel Oil, Peppermint Plant Oil, Ginger Root Oil, Cinnamon Bark Oil), Xylitol, Isomalt, Magnesium Stearate, Stevia, Citric Acid, Menthol

Slim & Sassy® Metabolic Gum

Slim & Sassy Metabolic Gum is yet another great way for you to get more of this wonderful essential oil blend into your daily routine.

Part Number: 60200347
Size: 32 Pieces   Wholesale: $8.50   Retail: $11.33   PV: 5

Click to Buy Now Slim & Sassy®: Metabolic Chewing Gum or Copy and Paste in Browser: http://bit.ly/2IEZ8V5

Description

Slim & Sassy metabolic oil blend helps manage cravings throughout the day while supporting healthy metabolism. There is one drop of Slim & Sassy essential oil blend in each piece of sugar-free gum. Slim & Sassy Metabolic Gum is yet another great way for you to get more of this wonderful essential oil blend into your daily routine.

Slim & Sassy essential oil blend contains Grapefruit, Lemon, Peppermint, Ginger, and Cinnamon. When taken internally with a healthy eating and exercise plan, Slim & Sassy Metabolic Blend can help you reach your weight management goals.

Uses

Chew one piece to help manage cravings throughout the day while supporting a healthy metabolism.

*These statements have not been evaluated by the Food and Drug Administration. This product is not intended to diagnose, treat, cure, or prevent any disease.

Slim & Sassy® TrimShakes Q & A

Are TrimShakes gluten, GMO, and soy free?

TrimShakes do not contain gluten, genetically modified material (GMO), or soy-based ingredients.

Does TrimShake contain sugar?

TrimShake does not contain evaporated cane juice or sugar. It is completely sweetened by stevia.

What are the natural flavors listed on the TrimShake label?

The natural flavors are a proprietary blend of natural flavors, including natural vanilla bean and cocoa flavors.

Is TrimShake a meal replacement?

TrimShake provides a healthy, low-fat, sugar free source of protein that delivers more than 20 vitamins, minerals, and other essential nutrients. TrimShake can be used several times daily to replace meals, snacks, or dessert, however, be sure to consume at least one well-balanced, nutritious meal daily.

What is Ashwagandha?

Ashwagandha is an herb native to India. It is included in TrimShake for its ability to help manage appetite and cravings.

How does an appetite suppressant work?

An appetite suppressant helps you feel fuller longer, or decreases the desire to eat.

Can I maintain the same benefits by adding fruits, juices, or vegetables to the TrimShakes?

Yes. Not only does it allow you to cater to your tastes by adding other things to your blender, but you can also add to an already robust list of nutrients.

Where can I find recipes of things other people have added to their TrimShakes?

Search for "TrimShakes" on doterra.com, or visit the product blog to see recipes like our TrimShake Fudgesicles, or Trimshake Granola Blueberry Crisp.

PRODUCT 4a

Slim & Sassy® TrimShakes – Vanilla Flavor

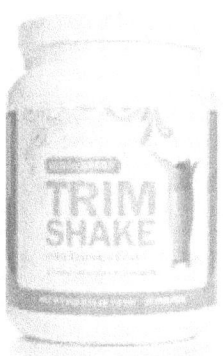

"For your meal replacement needs, Slim & Sassy TrimShake offers a very low calorie and sugar-free meal shake full of vital nutrients and fiber. TrimShake includes the patented ingredient EssentraTrim®†, which has been shown to assist in cortisol regulation. Also included is Solathin®†, a natural protein extract that supports a feeling a fullness.

Figure 3 TrimShake Has 2 Flavors, Vanilla & Chocolate. Presently Orange has been added on a temporary Basic

Blended with water or nonfat dairy, almond, soy, or rice milk, TrimShake offers a delicious and filling alternative to fast food when you need nutrition in a hurry. As a replacement for a full meal or as a delicious snack, Slim & Sassy TrimShake helps keep you satiated and helps maintain healthy blood glucose levels throughout the day so that you can focus on other components of your weight management plan." *Contributed by Damian Rodriguez, DHSc, MS*

Slim & Sassy® TrimShake—Chocolate

Primary Benefits

- Provides a convenient low-fat, low-sodium, low-calorie, sugar-free, lean alternative that is a good source of fiber for individuals trying to lose fat or maintain a lean body composition through calorie reduction and exercise
- Helps manage the release of the stress hormone cortisol, which is associated with the accumulation of fat, particularly around the stomach, hips, and thighs

44

- May help control stress-induced appetite, overeating, and carbohydrate cravings
- May help support blood sugar levels already in the normal range and enhance energy levels while helping to alleviate fatigue commonly associated with dieting and exercise

Slim & Sassy® TrimShake—Chocolate

For all chocolate lovers, Slim & Sassy Chocolate TrimShake is a low-calorie and delicious weight management mix created to help fight hunger cravings and enhance energy levels while alleviating fatigue.

Part Number: 35200001   Wholesale: $39.50   Retail: $52.67   PV: 25

Click to Buy Now: TrimShake –Chocolate
or Copy and Paste in Browser: http://bit.ly/2IEZ8V5

Description

dōTERRA Slim & Sassy TrimShake is a convenient and delicious weight management shake mix that provides essential nutrients and only 70 calories per serving. Blended with water or nonfat dairy, almond, rice, or soy milk, TrimShake can be used as part of a weight-loss strategy of reducing daily caloric intake and burning fat stores through exercise.

Slim & Sassy TrimShake includes the patented weight-loss ingredient EssentraTrim†, which research has shown to help manage cortisol—a stress hormone associated with fat storage in the abdomen, hips, and thighs. Slim & Sassy TrimShake also includes Solathin‡, a special protein extract from natural food sources that supports an increased feeling of satiety.

Available in natural chocolate and vanilla flavors, TrimShake blends well with water or milk and provides 8 grams of protein and 2.5 grams of fiber per serving.

† EssentraTrim® is a trademark of NutraGenesis LLC and is protected under U.S. Patent 6,713,092. ‡Solathin® is a trademark of CYVEX Nutrition

Uses

Blend one scoop of shake mix in ½ cup of water or nonfat dairy, almond, rice, or soy milk until smooth and creamy. Also, blends well with fruits and vegetables. For unique flavor options, blend one drop of your favorite dōTERRA essential oil in shake. Serve chilled.

*These statements have not been evaluated by the Food and Drug Administration. This product is not intended to diagnose, treat, cure, or prevent any disease.

PRODUCT 4b

Slim & Sassy® TrimShake—Orange Cream

(This Orange Product Is Available on a temporary Basic) Add to water, milk)

Slim & Sassy Orange Cream TrimShake is a low-calorie and delicious weight management mix created to help fight hunger cravings and enhance energy levels while alleviating fatigue. This product is only available for a limited-time.

Part Number: 60200657
Size: 640 G (40 Servings) Wholesale: $39.50   Retail: $52.67   PV: 25

Click to Buy Now: TrimShake –Orange Cream
or Copy and Paste in Browser: http://bit.ly/2IEZ8V5

Description

dōTERRA Slim & Sassy TrimShake is now available in an orange cream flavor! This convenient and delicious weight management shake mix provides essential nutrients and only 70 calories per serving.

Blended with water or nonfat dairy, almond, rice, or soy milk, TrimShake can be used as part of a weight-loss strategy of reducing daily caloric intake and burning fat stores through exercise.

Slim & Sassy TrimShake includes the patented weight-loss ingredient EssentraTrim[†], which, research has shown, helps manage cortisol—a stress hormone associated with fat storage in the abdomen, hips, and thighs.

Slim & Sassy TrimShake also includes Solathin[‡], a special protein extract from natural food sources that supports an increased feeling of satiety. TrimShake blends well with water or milk and provides 8 grams of protein and 2.5 grams of fiber per serving.

†EssentraTrim® is a trademark of NutraGenesis LLC and is protected under U.S. Patent 6,713,092 ‡Solathin® is a trademark of CYVEX Nutrition

Uses

Blend one scoop of shake mix in ½ cup of water or nonfat dairy, almond, rice, or soy milk until smooth and creamy. Also, blends well with fruits and vegetables. For unique flavor options, blend one drop of your favorite dōTERRA essential oil in shake. Serve chilled.

Primary Benefits

- Provides a convenient low-fat, low-sodium, low-calorie, sugar-free, lean alternative that is a good source of fiber for individuals trying to lose fat or maintain a lean body composition through calorie reduction and exercise.
- Helps manage the release of the stress hormone cortisol, which is associated with the accumulation of fat, particularly around the stomach, hips, and thighs
- May help control stress-induced appetite, overeating, and carbohydrate cravings
- May help support blood sugar levels already in the normal range and enhance energy levels while helping to alleviate fatigue commonly associated with dieting and exercise

*These statements have not been evaluated by the Food and Drug Administration. This product is not intended to diagnose, treat, cure, or prevent any disease.

PRODUCT 4c

Slim & Sassy® TrimShake—Vanilla
Add to water, milk, one compete meal replacement.

Primary Benefits

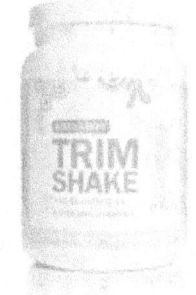

- Provides a convenient low-fat, low-sodium, low-calorie, sugar-free, lean alternative that is a good source of fiber for individuals trying to lose fat or maintain a lean body composition through calorie reduction and exercise

Figure 4
TrimShake—Vanilla

- Helps manage the release of the stress hormone cortisol, which is associated with the accumulation of fat, particularly around the stomach, hips, and thighs
- May help control stress-induced appetite, overeating, and carbohydrate cravings
- May help support blood sugar levels already in the normal range and enhance energy levels while helping to alleviate fatigue commonly associated with dieting and exercise

Slim & Sassy® TrimShake—Vanilla

dōTERRA Slim & Sassy Vanilla TrimShake is a tasty weight management shake mix. Trimshake is low-calorie and provides essential nutrients.

Part Number: 35180001   Wholesale: $39.50   Retail: $52.67   PV: 25

Click to Buy Now: TrimShake –Vanilla
or Copy and Paste in Browser: http://bit.ly/2lEZ8V5

Description

dōTERRA Slim & Sassy TrimShake is a convenient and delicious weight management shake mix that provides essential nutrients and only 70 calories per serving. Blended with water or nonfat dairy, almond, rice, or soy milk, TrimShake can be used as part of a weight-loss strategy of reducing daily caloric intake and burning fat stores through exercise.

Slim & Sassy TrimShake includes the patented weight-loss ingredient EssentraTrim†, which research has shown to help manage cortisol—a stress hormone associated with fat storage in the abdomen, hips, and thighs.

Slim & Sassy TrimShake also includes Solathin‡, a special protein extract from natural food sources that supports an increased feeling of satiety.

Available in natural chocolate and vanilla flavors, TrimShake blends well with water or milk and provides 8 grams of protein and 2.5 grams of fiber per serving.

† EssentraTrim® is a trademark of NutraGenesis LLC and is protected under U.S. Patent 6,713,092

‡Solathin® is a trademark of CYVEX Nutrition

Uses

Blend one scoop of shake mix in ½ cup of water or nonfat dairy, almond, rice, or soy milk until smooth and creamy. Also, blends well with fruits and vegetables. For unique flavor options, blend one drop of your favorite dōTERRA essential oil in shake. Serve chilled.

*These statements have not been evaluated by the Food and Drug Administration. This product is not intended to diagnose, treat, cure, or prevent any disease.

Slim & Sassy® (Vegetarian) V Shake Q & A

Does the Slim & Sassy® V Shake contain gluten?

Slim & Sassy V shake does not contain gluten or gluten-containing ingredients, nor was it produced in a facility that processes gluten-containing grains.

Does the Slim & Sassy® V Shake contain GMOs?

Nothing in the Slim & Sassy V shake contain Genetically Modified Material (GMO).

Does the Slim & Sassy® V Shake contain soy or dairy?

Slim & Sassy V Shake does not contain soy or soy-derived ingredients, nor does it contain any dairy-derived ingredients.

Is it safe for my child to take the Slim & Sassy® V Shake?

It is not recommended that children use Slim & Sassy V Shake to replace meals. However, Slim & Sassy V Shake is safe for children to use as a snack at a one scoop dose if desired.

What is the difference between the Slim & Sassy® V Shake and TrimShake?

Slim & Sassy V Shake is an entirely vegan alternative to Slim & Sassy TrimShake. It can be used in place of Slim & Sassy TrimShake as a meal replacement or weight loss aid for adults that want to get the benefits of Slim & Sassy TrimShake but prefer a vegan alternative.

Is Slim & Sassy® V Shake just as effective for weight management as Slim & Sassy TrimShake?

Slim & Sassy V Shake contains a similar amount of protein and calories as Slim & Sassy TrimShake, so it can be used as an aid for weight management in the same way Slim & Sassy TrimShake is used.

PRODUCT 5
Slim & Sassy® (Vegetarian) V Shake

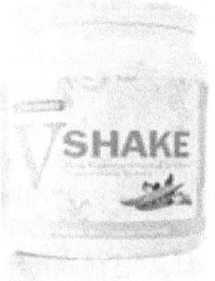

Primary Benefits

- Each serving contains 7 grams of protein from a proprietary vegan blend of pea, amaranth, and quinoa protein; contains no soy.
- Each serving includes 125 mg EssentraTrim®, a patented extract of ashwagandha leaves and roots clinically studied to help control the release of the stress hormone cortisol, which is associated with the accumulation of fat, particularly around the stomach, hips, and thighs.
- Each serving includes 50 mg of Solathin, a special protein extract from natural food sources that supports an increased feeling of satiety.

Figure 5: Figure 5Slim & Sassy Vegetarian Shake

Slim & Sassy® V Shake

Part Number: 35440001   Wholesale: $39.50   Retail: $52.67   PV: 25

Click to Buy Now: Slim & Sassy® V Shake
or Copy and Paste in Browser: http://bit.ly/2IEZ8V5

Description

dōTERRA Slim & Sassy V Shake is a convenient, completely vegan-friendly, delicious weight management shake mix that provides essential nutrients and only 74 calories per serving.

V Shake can be used as part of a weight-loss strategy of reducing daily calorie intake and burning fat stores through exercise. Slim & Sassy V Shake includes the patented weight-loss ingredient EssentraTrim, which has been clinically studied to help manage cortisol—a stress hormone associated with fat storage in the abdomen, hips, and thighs.

Slim & Sassy V Shake also includes Solathin, a special protein extract from natural food sources that supports an increased feeling of satiety. V Shake blends well with water or rice, soy or almond milk and provides 7 grams of protein and 4 grams of fiber per serving.

Uses

Blend one scoop of shake mix in 1/2 cup of almond, rice, or soy milk, or water until smooth

and creamy. Also, blends well with fruits and vegetables. For unique flavor options, blend one drop of your favorite dōTERRA essential oil in shake. Serve chilled.

Does not contain artificial sweeteners, flavors, colors, or preservatives.

† EssentraTrim® is a trademark of NutraGenesis LLC and is protected under U.S. Patent 6,713,092

‡Solathin® is a trademark of CYVEX Nutrition

PRODUCT 6

Slim & Sassy® New You Kit Includes Free Membership

Buy a kit and get a FREE one year membership with any KIT. You also get 25% discount on any purchase **X** one year. When you purchase any kit, you get a bonus of a   membership. This is a $35.00 value good for 12 months.

Slim & Sassy® New You Kit

Combined with exercise and healthy eating, the Slim & Sassy New You Kit can help with weight management and can assist in curbing cravings, promoting a healthy metabolism, and enhancing energy. *

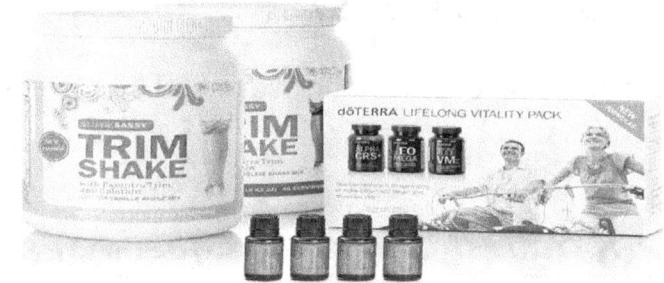

Figure 6: New You Kit with Free Membership

Part Number: 41360001   Wholesale: $199.00   Retail: $265.33   PV: 150

Description

Be ready with all the products you need for the next Slim and Sassy Lifestyle Change Competition with the Slim & Sassy New You Kit. Reach your goals and slim down by using Slim & Sassy on a regular basis throughout the day along with doTERRA TrimShakes and the doTERRA Lifelong Vitality Pack®. Slim & Sassy New You Kit includes four Slim & Sassy 15 mL metabolic blends, one vanilla and one chocolate TrimShake (40 servings), and the Lifelong Vitality Pack.

*These statements have not been evaluated by the Food and Drug Administration. This product is not intended to diagnose, treat, cure, or prevent any disease.

Click to Buy Now: Slim & Sassy® New You Kit
or Copy and Paste in Browser: http://bit.ly/2IEZ8V5

Description

Be ready with all the products you need for the next Slim and Sassy Lifestyle Change Competition with the Slim & Sassy New You Kit. Reach your goals and slim down by using

Slim & Sassy on a regular basis throughout the day along with dōTERRA TrimShakes and the dōTERRA Lifelong Vitality Pack®. Slim & Sassy New You Kit includes four Slim & Sassy 15 mL metabolic blends, one vanilla and one chocolate TrimShake (40 servings), and the Lifelong Vitality Pack.

PRODUCT 7

Slim & Sassy® Trim Kit - 1 Chocolate, 1 Vanilla

Combined to give a kick-start to a healthier life, Slim & Sassy Trim Kit contains Slim & Sassy Metabolic Blends and TrimShake mixes to help fight hunger cravings, support a healthy metabolism, and promote increased energy levels.

Part Number: 40770001
Size: Four 15 mL bottles of Slim & Sassy Metabolic Blend and two TrimShakes
Wholesale: $150.00   Retail: $200.00   PV: 125

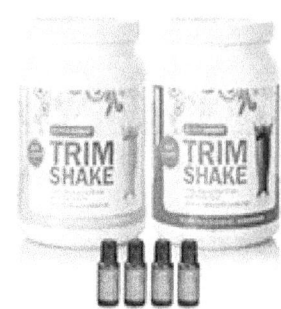

Figure 7Slim & Sassy® Trim Kit - 1 Chocolate, 1 Vanilla

Click to Buy Now: 1 Chocolate, 1 Vanilla
or Copy and Paste in Browser: http://bit.ly/2IEZ8V5

Description

Kick off your weight management goals with the Slim & Sassy Trim Kit. Slim down by using Slim & Sassy Metabolic Blend in your water, or use topically, throughout the day as part of your new commitment to improve your lifestyle with diet and exercise. Reduce your cravings with satisfying TrimShakes. This kit includes:

- Four 15 mL bottles Slim & Sassy Metabolic Blend
- 1 Chocolate TrimShake (40 servings) & 1 Vanilla TrimShake (40 servings)

PRODUCT 8

Slim & Sassy® Trim Kit - 2 Chocolate Trim Shakes

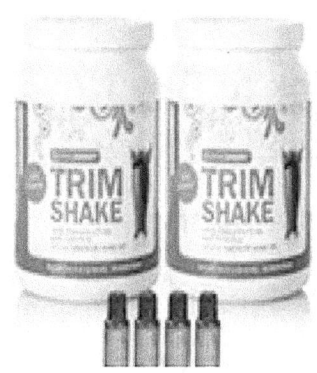

Combined to give a kick-start to a healthier life, Slim & Sassy Trim Kit contains Slim & Sassy Metabolic Blends and TrimShake mixes to help fight hunger cravings, support a healthy metabolism, and promote increased energy levels.

Part Number: 35280001
Size: Four 15 mL bottles of Slim & Sassy Metabolic Blend and two TrimShakes. Wholesale: $150.00   Retail: $200.00   PV: 125

Figure 8: Slim & Sassy® Trim Kit - 2 Chocolate Trim Shakes

Click to Buy Now: Slim & Sassy® Trim Kit - 2 Chocolate Trim Shakes. or Copy and Paste URL in Browser: http://bit.ly/2IEZ8V5

Description

Kick off your weight management goals with the Slim & Sassy Trim Kit. Slim down by using Slim & Sassy Metabolic Blend in your water, or use topically, throughout the day as part of your new commitment to improve your lifestyle with diet and exercise. Reduce your cravings with satisfying TrimShakes. This kit includes:

- Four 15 mL bottles Slim & Sassy Metabolic Blend
- Two Chocolate TrimShakes (40 servings each)

PRODUCT 9

Slim & Sassy® Trim Kit - 2 Vanilla Trim Shakes

Combined to give a kick-start to a healthier life, Slim & Sassy Trim Kit contains Slim & Sassy Metabolic Blends and TrimShake mixes to help fight hunger cravings, support a healthy metabolism, and promote increased energy levels.

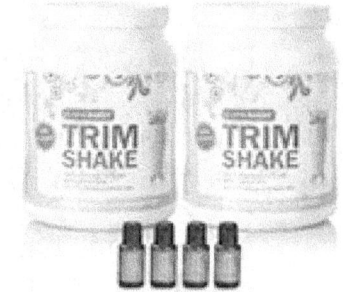

Part Number: 35290001
Size: Four 15 mL bottles of Slim & Sassy Metabolic Blend and two TrimShakes. Wholesale: $150.00   Retail: $200.00   PV: 125

Figure 9Slim & Sassy® Trim Kit - 2 Vanilla Trim Shakes

Click to Buy Now: Slim & Sassy® Trim Kit - 2 Vanilla Trim Shakes. or Copy and Paste URL in Browser: https://bitly.com/#

Description

Kick off your weight management goals with the Slim & Sassy Trim Kit. Slim down by using Slim & Sassy Metabolic Blend in your water, or use topically, throughout the day as part of your new commitment to improve your lifestyle with diet and exercise. Reduce your cravings with satisfying TrimShakes. This kit includes:

- Four 15 mL bottles Slim & Sassy Metabolic Blend
- Two Vanilla TrimShakes (40 servings each)

PRODUCT 10

Slim & Sassy® Trim Kit—2 V Shake

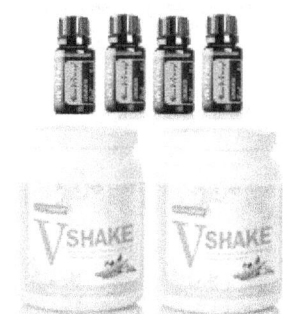

Part Number: 60130001
Size: Four 15 mL bottles of Slim & Sassy Metabolic Blend and two TrimShakes

Wholesale: $150.00   Retail: $200.00   PV: 125

Figure 10 Slim & Sassy®
Trim Kit—2 V Shake

Click Here to Buy Now: Slim & Sassy® Trim Kit—2 V Shake

or Copy and Paste URL in Browser: http://bit.ly/2IEZ8V5

Description

Introducing a vegetarian alternative to weight management shakes. Slim & Sassy V Shake provides the same benefits as TrimShake except for all the ingredients being 100 percent plant-sourced and vegetarian-friendly.

Includes:

Four 15 mL Slim & Sassy Metabolic Blend, Two V Shakes.

PRODUCT 11

The dōTERRA Lifelong Vitality Pack®, including Alpha CRS®+, XEO Mega®, and Microplex MVp™

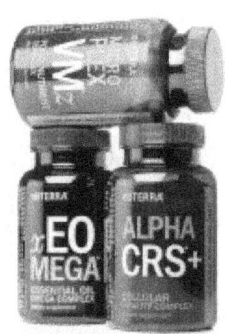

Lifelong Vitality Supplements
New Lifelong Vitality Pack
LRP Only (Means must have a membership to purchase this one)   *Figure 11 Lifelong Vitality Pack*

dōTERRA's Lifelong Vitality supplements are formulated with potent levels of essential nutrients and powerful metabolic factors for optimal health, energy, and longevity.

Coupled with dōTERRA's CPTG Certified Pure Therapeutic Grade essential oils and a lifelong commitment to dōTERRA's wellness lifestyle, they naturally support a lifetime of looking, feeling and living younger, longer.

Note: This pack and its personalized components are available only at enrollment or when added to a new or existing Loyalty Reward order. Get this kit at:

| #d20640001 | Your Price $79.50 | Retail $106.00 | PV 60 |

Click to buy now: Lifelong Vitality Kit

or Copy URL and put in Browser: http://bit.ly/2IEZ8V5

The dōTERRA Lifelong Vitality Pack®, including Alpha CRS®+, XEO Mega®, and Microplex MVp™ is the next component of healthy weight management. * Formulated to provide your body with essential nutrients and powerful metabolic factors for lifelong wellness, they are even more crucial when on a calorie-restricted diet. *

When reducing caloric intake, even if you are basing your nutrition choices on whole, nutrient-dense foods, you will inherently have a greater risk for nutrient deficiencies. Being in a negative energy balance also generally leaves people feeling sluggish, which can affect their physical activity habits and mood. dōTERRA Lifelong Vitality Pack addresses both these issues, along with supporting healthy metabolism. *

The potent antioxidant and energy cofactors in Alpha CRS+ support natural energy production without the use of stimulants. * The combination of essential fatty acids in xEO Mega support healthy immune function, an important factor when on a calorie-restricted nutrition plan. * Lastly, MicroPlex MVp Food Nutrient Complex provides a highly bioavailable source of vitamins and minerals, some of which are commonly deficient in modern and calorie-restricted diets. The products included in the dōTERRA Lifelong Vitality Pack work synergistically to provide you with key nutrients and the energy and immune support you need to remain healthy when cutting calories. *

Helping to maintain satiety, minimize toxic load, manage stress, and support your body's natural metabolism, supplementing with dōTERRA Slim & Sassy products and the dōTERRA Lifelong Vitality Pack provides the foundation for a successful weight management plan. * Following the healthy lifestyle pyramid, sustainable weight management is within your reach. * *Contributed by Damian Rodriguez, DHSc, MS*

If you struggle with weight like many, you've probably figured out what scientists and doctors already know: that there is no magic weight loss pill. We just can't keep eating too much and exercising too little and then expect a pill to fix it.

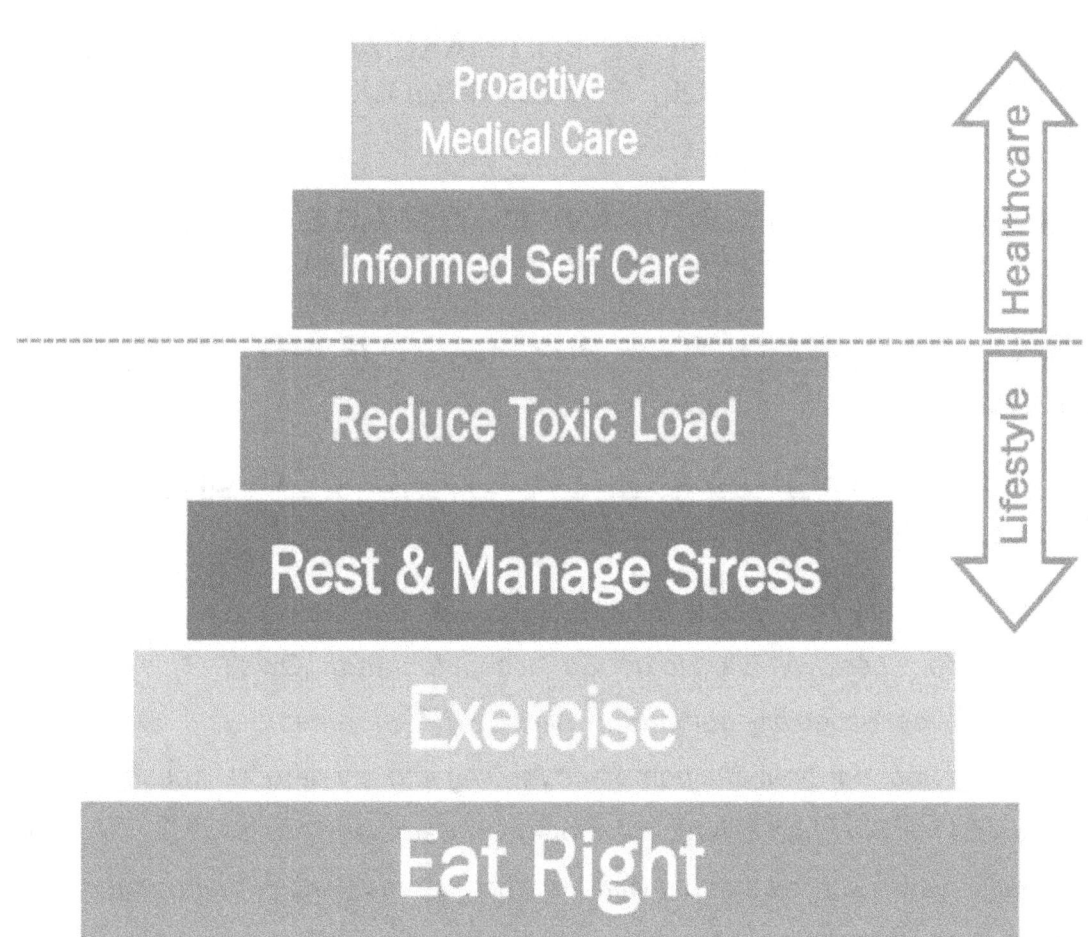

Successful weight loss requires lifestyle improvements. Weight management is right at the foundation of dōTERRA Wellness Lifestyle, and if you like it or not, it involves eating right and exercising. These lifestyle improvements need to be long-term changes to really get lasting results. I know you have a winner in you because God created you a winner.

Our current Slim & Sassy program already provides excellent products and tools to help people reach their goals, including the Slim & Sassy Metabolic essential oil blend and our high-protein Trim Shakes.

1. **GET A MEMBERSHIP BEFORE YOU MAKE A PURCHASE TODAY.** RECEIVE INSTANT 25% OFF EVERY PRODUCT PURCHASED FOR 12 FULL MONTHS.

2. **MEMBERSHIP IS FREE WITH ANY OF THE KITS PURCHASED** A $35.00 GIFT TO YOU. Yes, Membership has its benefits!

3. **CLICK HERE TO MAKE YOUR PURCHASE OF ANY OF THE PRODUCTS.**

4. **SEE ALL THE WEIGHT MANAGEMENT PRODUCTS ON ONE PAGE, CLICK HERE.**

5. *"You are completely responsible for where you are, just like you are completely responsible for where you want to go. So, accept that truth. Own it. This concept has defined our lives, especially our journey in dōTERRA. I remember when we were driving away from our beautiful home and moving into my parents' house—I felt depressed. I felt like I had fallen behind on my dreams and "it wasn't fair." A short time later, my wife shared a quote with me from Dennis Waitley that opened our hearts to a new possibility:*

   "There are two primary choices in life, to accept conditions as they exist or accept responsibility for changing them." Tell yourself: "If I got myself in this, I can get myself out." I have noticed time and time again that those who succeed look for the circumstances that they want, and if they can't find them, they create them. But, probably the hardest part of getting to this point is recognizing that your strategies and your behavior patterns are not working. Sometimes this means that you need to reinvent yourself, but you have the power to do so."

BONUSES START HERE

When I monitored my own health and healthcare, I have discovered that I become what I eat. I become what I think. My results are equaled to my efforts.

There's no short cut to achieving your goals, dreams or ambitions without first putting in the work. You can lose weight and keep it off too. You will too with effort.

Overweight and obesity is becoming a worldwide pandemic because most people want the quick fix solution. I will stop planning, purchasing the products to prepare most of my meals. Instead I will drink extra-large sugary drinks, eat fast foods everyday, refused to exercise regularly and be healthy everyday.

But our beautiful, wonderful bodies don't function that way. We only get from it, what we feed it with. Junk foods in, disease out. Or quality nutrients in, vibrant health out. Some get the bonus of a long and happy life.

THEREFORE, CONSIDERING THIS FACT, OUR TEAM HAVE PREPARED FOR YOU SOME RELEVANT INFORMATION TO HELP YOU LOSE WEIGHT EVERYDAY AND KEEP IT OFF.

THE WEIGHT LOSS INDUSTRY SELLS BILLIONS OF USELESS PRODUCTS TO FOOL MANY THAT THEY CAN LOSE WEIGHT AND KEEP IT OFF. INSTEAD, OVERWEIGHT AND OBESITY IS ALMOST A PANDEMIC...

GOVERNMENTS SPEND 6 TRILLION DOLLARS YEARLY FIGHTING THE LIFESTYLE DISEASES...YET PEOPLE ARE DYING AT AN EARLY AGE AND OBESITY EXPLODES.

USE THESE BONUSES TO LEARN HOW TO LOSE WEIGHT EVERYDAY AND KEEP IT OFF.

BONUS # 1

The Proper Definition To Lose Weight

Losing weight takes effort, time, energy, and will power to get that perfect weight and figure you've always dreamed of. Before going to the **proper** step-by-step of how-to's, let us first warm our minds up on the right information about losing weight everyday. What's the real deal, anyway?

Is Health Wealth?

Wealth can be a temporary thing as many people are discovering. Whether from the housing bust or from financial loss via hurricanes, fires or floods, becoming wealthy is not about acquiring all the riches in the world nor getting whatever you want at a snap of the fingers. It's more about investing something from an earlier period of your life and being able to continuously use it perfectly until you grow old. No material thing can be such an investment because one day they come, and before you know it, they go. For instance, the money you saved today may be the insurance for heart surgery due to obesity complications later in your life. Or medications for pain due to body aches from lifestyle diseases.

There is no guarantee that the money you earned from hard work will be just for fun and security. If you are sick and have money are you healthy? If you have lots of money but very sick, are you wealthy?

The real richness in this world is being happy, contented, and satisfied – being able to do what you want to do, when you want to do it. How can you truly enjoy the soda drinks if you know that it is increasing your weight which is causing you knee pain? How can you enjoy a pint of ice cream if you're not allowed to eat it because you're diabetic? Or what good is a big house that you live in when most of the time of your life you are in a hospital because of serious lifestyle illnesses? In other words, money, riches, and other classy material things are no good at all when you can't even enjoy them, eat them, or simply have them because certain sicknesses forbid you to, isn't it sad?

What's better is not having any allergy to animal furs even if you can't afford to buy a pet, not being diabetic even if a scoop of ice cream will do for dessert, and staying in your own house even if it's not so big to fit 3 people inside. When you are healthy and in perfect shape, lack, or even absence, of material resources will not matter anymore. As long as you can do whatever you want to do, eat whatever your tongue feels like eating, and go wherever your feet brings you to, you'll never be more contented in your life; thus, making you wealthier than any rich-but-sick people out there.

Healthy People What Did They Get?

People who are considered "healthy" are those who are physically and mentally fit. Physical fitness is the ability of the human body to function with vigor and alertness. Also, without undue fatigue, with ample energy to engage in leisure activities, and to meet physical stresses. Muscular strength, endurance, stamina, and general alertness are the overt signs of being physically fit.

The level of physical fitness can be influenced by regular, systematic exercise and proper nutrition. Moderate activity will maintain the individual at a level that is usually adequate to handle ordinary stress, while right diet affects energy expenditure. Overweight, underweight, and weak individuals have low fitness levels.

On the other hand, mental fitness refers to the psychological state of well-being, characterized by continuing personal growth, a sense of purpose in life, self-acceptance, and positive relations with others.

Obesity Leads To Unhealthy People

In contrast with the above discussion, people who belong to the "unhealthy" category are the opposite of the healthy ones. They are unwell either in the body or in the mind, or in both. Physically, they are ill or they show symptoms of ill health. These sicknesses hinder them from performing daily activities properly. They get easily fatigued or stressed resulting in unaccomplished tasks. Absence, lack, or inappropriate exercise and food intake is what makes people physically unfit.

Alternatively, one can also be mentally unhealthy if his psychological state is not well. Manifestations include always being doubtful, worries too much, suffers from inferiority complex, relates negatively to others or using foods for comfort seeking…

How to Rate Your Weight?
The Normal Way: Height-Weight Relationship

Physical health can be measured through the appropriateness of a person's weight to his height. This is done where the body weight refers to the measure of one's heaviness, and the height is the measure of his tallness.

1. **Example:** A woman measuring 5 ft high (1.52 m), with a medium body frame should weigh between 103 lbs to 115 lbs (46.72 kg – 52.16 kg) to be considered healthy.

2. **Another example:** A man standing 5 ft 8 in (1.72 m) tall, with a large body frame is healthy if he is weighing between 144 lbs – 163 lbs (65.32 kg – 73.94 kg).

Otherwise, if their weight is lower than the desired body weight for their height, they are considered underweight, and if, in turn, their weight is higher than the desired body weight for their height, they are said to be overweight. (See Appendix A: Desirable eight Ranges).

Body Mass Index (BMI)

Body Mass Index is an accurate indicator of surplus body fat than kilos or pounds. It is a mathematical ratio of height to weight that can be linked with body composition (or body fat percentage) and with indices of health risk.

Calculating BMI is as follows:

$$BMI = \frac{\text{Weight (in kg)}}{\text{Height (in m)}^2} \qquad \text{or} \qquad BMI = \frac{\text{Weight (in lbs) x 700}}{\text{Height (in inches)}^2}$$

Example, the calculation for someone weighing 80 kg (176 lbs) and 1.60 m (63 in) tall is:

$$BMI = \frac{80}{160^2} = 31.2 \qquad \text{or} \qquad BMI = \frac{176 \times 700}{63^2} = 31.1$$

People with a BMI of 25.1 to 29.9 are considered overweight, and people with a BMI of 30 or above are considered obese. Thus, from the example above, a person weighing 80 kg and is 1.60 m tall is obese. A high BMI assumes a higher percentage of body fat, which places a person at greater risk for developing chronic diseases and other serious illnesses.

BMI	Weight Category
Under 19	Underweight
20-25	Normal (Healthy)
26-30	Overweight
30 above	Obese

Table 1.1 Body Weight Categories According to BMI

However, for some people, the BMI is not a reliable indication of health. A highly muscled individual who is very fit and healthy may have a somewhat heavy body weight because muscles pack on a lot of pounds. This person may have a high BMI that improperly puts him or her in the overweight or obese categories. Likewise, thin individuals who have a low body weight with very little muscle and a higher percentage of fat may have a normal BMI, which would be an incorrect indication of healthiness.

Support for Obesity

Obesity is defined as being 20 percent or more above one's desirable weight range (See appendix A again for reference). It is a medical condition that refers primarily to storage of excess body fat. The human body naturally stores fat tissue under the skin and around organs and joints. Fat is critical for good health because it is a source of energy when the body lacks natural energy necessary to sustain life processes. It also provides insulation and protection for internal organs.

The accumulation of too much fat in the body is associated with a variety of health problems. The person who is obese needs encouragment to put in place certain selfcontrol to manage eating proper foods, avoid sugary drinks, fatty foods, limit junk and fast foods. Exercise at least 30 minutes per day, four to five days per week. You can do this!

Causes of Obesity

A calorie is the unit used to measure the energy value of food and the energy used by the body to maintain normal functions. When the calories from food intake equal the calories of energy the body uses, weight remains constant. But when more calories are eaten than the body needs, the body stores those additional calories as fat, causing subsequent weight gain. <u>One pound (1 lb) of fat represents about 3,500 excess calories</u>.

Obesity is partially determined by a person's genetic makeup. If a child inherited the excessive body fat cells of his obese parents, more likely, he will tend to eat more than his body needs; thus, making him obese too. Copying poor eating habits of parents also affects a child's body weight.

Lifestyles also play a key role in triggering obesity. Eating big servings of food at restaurants and fast foods more frequently than nutritious home-cooked foods could help adding more calories and fats rather than limiting them. Devoting less time for exercise and other physical activities do not control weight gain. And doing untiring recreational activities such as browsing the internet, video games, movies, and television, plus using laborsaving devices of the modern living, such as personal computers, telephones, and remote controls, promote an inactive lifestyle.

Effects and Possible Complications of Obesity

Obesity Increases the Risk of Developing Disease.

According to some studies, almost 70 percent of heart disease cases in the United States are linked to excess body fat. Obese people are more than twice as likely to develop high blood pressure. Obese women are twice at risk for developing breast cancer, and all obese people have an estimated 42 percent higher chance of developing colon cancer. Almost 80 percent of patients with Type 2, or non-insulin-dependent diabetes mellitus are obese. The risk of medical complications, particularly heart disease, increases when body fat is distributed around the waist, especially in the abdomen. This type of upper body fat distribution is more common in men than in women.

The social and psychological problems experienced by obese people are also challenging. Discrimination for "fat" people is most likely to occur in educational institutions, employment, and social relationships. Other psychological effects include stress, nervous tension, boredom, frustration, lack of friends, depression, inferiority complex, and poor self-esteem.

There are a few tips to keep in mind as you start the "30-Day Lose Weight Plan" using the Natural Appetite-control Products & Supplements - NAPS. Dilute with dōTERRA's Fractionated Coconut Oil to minimize any skin sensitivity.

More Health Complications of Obesity

Heart disease, High blood pressure, Cancer (Some cancer), Addiction, Balance, Diabetes, Strokes, Gallbladder disease, Breathing problems, Bloating and stomach upsets, Varicose veins, Kidney disease, Psychological effects include, stress, nervous tension, boredom, frustration, lack of friends, depression, lacks confidence, self control, panic attack, fear, inferiority complex, and poor self-esteem.

Did you know what the survey said...

- Worldwide the obesity rate has more than doubled since the 1980s.

- Recent research states: more than 1.9 billion adults, 18 years and older, were overweight. Of these over 600 million were obese. Obesity is preventable.

- 39% of adults over 18 years were overweight in 2014, and 13% were obese.

- Most of the world's population live in countries where overweight and obesity kills more people than underweight.

- 41 million children under the age of 5 were overweight or obese in 2014.

BONUS # 2

The Proper Plan To Lose Weight

Before taking actions in any problem we encounter, there should always be a plan first. That is, if we want to come up with positive results. You wouldn't want to enter a battle without preparing how to defeat the enemy, would you? Operating a task without planning is like building a house without a blueprint or fighting against a basketball team without a team play with your teammates. How would you expect a good outcome?

Imagine this too, building the house without submitting the blueprint to the county office for proper zoning and regulations checks. That's no different, when we refuse to call in the big guys. It is Jesus, His Father, God and the Holy Spirit. We build in vain, we live in vain and die in vain. Losing weight is not at all different from the above mentioned plan-necessity situations. It also involves taking actions and proper ways that need to be perfectly planned in order to bring satisfying results. Nothing is too hard for God!

Setting Your Weight Goal

Because you now have Natural Appetite-control Products & Supplements - NAPS, you will have the help you previously lacked to lose weight. It is Okay to set your weight goal. Say your weight is 20% above the considered normal for your height, you tend to eat more than 5 regular meals a day. You're certain that you're physically unfit. Now, the question is, what do you want to happen?

Setting a goal is the first step in planning your future weight. Know what you want to accomplish. This way, the road you are taking is clear. You can keep track of your journey – whether or not you are going along the right direction. With a goal in mind, you are always motivated to finish a task, or in some cases, to start doing it. See Appendix B for your copy of the Lose Weight Everyday Weekly Diary to keep track of your progress.

Be Definite

Setting a specific goal, when planning to lose weight, improves your chances of success. Only, be clear and be definite with what you want to happen. Vague aims such as 'I'd like to be healthier' or 'I need to lose a few kilos,' tend to produce half-hearted efforts and very poor results. Instead, state your goal distinctly: 'I want to lose 2-3 kilos this week and every week' or 'I will trim my waist line from 40" down to 32" by the end of the month.' If you need to, write it down and put it where you will always see and read it. This way, you'll always be reminded of what you want and need to accomplish by the end of the month, the week, or even the day.

But imagine this. When you invite God into your planning, ask of Him to come into your goal setting and achieving, then you start to work as if you know you cannot fail, amazing things start to happen in your situation. Your unwillingness to exercise, start to change to willingness. Your taste buds starts to reject the sugary, salty, fatty foods too. I can only say boldly, when you start to "Live-life Under Christ Knowledge – LUCK", change takes place. Peace spring forth in your heart. Love abound and satisfaction is your joy. Do not rob yourself of abundant health by God. Make the call to the BIG guys today. It is Jesus, His Holy Father, God and The Holy Spirit.

Be Realistic

In establishing a definite weight goal, make sure that it is possible and doable – realistic, in simpler terms. How can a goal like 'I'll lose 15 lbs in just a week' happen if even the most accurate weight-loss diet suggests that you can only burn 6-7 lbs in a week? That is, if you follow strictly what the diet recommends. Weight loss goals need to be sensible so that it won't be far from coming true. What happens when you set a goal and it didn't happen, no matter how hard you tried because it wasn't really achievable in the first place? Here is what some people do. They get depressed, discouraged and disappointed which are some of the psychological causes of obesity. And the problem just goes in circles without really an end to it. So, many goes right back to eating even more addictive foods.

Do Not Punish Yourself – Plan Ahead

There is a tracking, Appendix B for you to write down your weight loss goal or what you want to achieve and keep it in an area you can see it. The next step is planning on how to accomplish it. Planning involves proper scheduling of activities to be done throughout the whole day for a certain period of time including exercises, meals, the TrimShakes and if you will subsitute a meal with on Trimshake. Track your sleeping and waking. It comprises of the time these activities should be done, the duration, and in the case of eating meals, the food to be consumed. This way, inappropriate spur-of-the-moments decisions can be avoided. <u>Be organized with this process as you really would like to break had habbits and reinvent yourself with good new habbits.</u>

Proper and effective plan consists of quality time for performing such activities. That is, ample and enough time. Plan to read the daily emails from the "30-Day Lose Weight Plan" These are the 30-day inspirationals to help you lose weight everyday.

Research suggests that it takes between eighteen to twenty-seven days to form a habbit. You will receive 30-days of supporting help and most of the products has a 30 days supply of products. Therefore, you have the extra days to help you break-in your new life using NAPS. Your are never alone as you will be encouraged to "Live-life Under Christ

Knowledge – LUCK. For example, sleep should be scheduled to last for around 7 to 8 hours a day so that you'll be able to get enough rest. Lack of sleep may cause improper eating habit the next day. Some people get two flavors of the TrimShake so they alternate and add fruits, vegetables, nuts or your favorites.

Again, plans should be relatively realistic. Include only time and activities you know for yourself you can accomplish for a given period of time. Also, as you finished preparing the plan, you might want to write it down since you can't always keep that it mind. Post it in a place where you can always see and read it to remind you what your plans are for the day. Try your best not to skip anything in your scheduled plan so as not to ruin the effectivity of it. Remember, your health depends on this plan. Do it right. Plan according to the examples above. Remember that trusting God, sleeping, exercise, and meals are the most essential elements to include in your daily schedule. Take note of the calorie intakes (through foods) and calorie burning (through exercises) for efficient results.

The Role of Positive Thinking

The earlier mentioned goals like "I'll lose 3 kilos this week," or "I'll trim my waist line down by 10 inches" are examples of affirmations. <u>Affirmations are positive thoughts that when truly believed will somehow help in making things happen</u>. Positive thinking produces positive reality by trigerring our body to do what it says; thus, providing you with will power. For example, if you truly believed that you will lose 3 kilos this week, your brain will command your body to do things this week in order to lose 3 kilos until it happens.

If you are not a positive person, this is the time to start positive affirmations. Positive statements about yourself or your intentions, are a deceptively simple aid to achieving this weight loss goal or anything you want to achieve. They work by imprinting themselves upon the subconscious mind through regular repetition – saying, reading, or writing them down over and over again. Some people even record their affirmations on audio and listen to them repeatedly to make sure that the thoughts are planted on the mind.

If you truly believe your affirmations and intend for them to come true, then they will. They do require a little discipline, but their benefits will surely outweigh the time and effort you spent. Remember, you become what you think. <u>God is on your side, you cannot fail</u>.

STOP DEPENDENCY ON SUGAR, SALT & FATS

You can stop your dependency on sugar, salt and fats that gives you a short rush of 'feeling good' and be uplifted for a few seconds of the day.

Today, I bring you sources and resources that will bring you out of your insufficiency into sufficiency. From sick, overweight and obese into slim, fit and sassy.

From poor self-esteem, into confidence in who you are and whose you are. Know this one thing, God has handpicked you to start a break out in you that no sugar, salt or fat can quench. He is about to melt the plaque blocking fats that fill your body and start the healthy alternative in your body, mind, spirit, emotions and finance. People will want to be around you. When you open your mouth, nothing but good uplifting words will come forth that will edify others. You will become contagious because everybody will want what you have. Start your "30-Day Lose Weight Plan" today and come learn.

Do not be afraid to be acquainted with God and His plan for your life. You are a winner and you will show others how to become a winner in this life and for eternity.

BONUS # 3

The Proper Diet To Lose Weight

For most of us, eating is one of the most enjoyable things we do in our everyday lives. How sad though, that one of the nicest things can cause many a young person to go to an early grave because of overweight and obesity. As a matter of fact, we have our favorite dishes, favorite sugary drinks, and favorite fast foods which only prove that eating is one of our favorite activities. There's really nothing wrong with that since food, is a primary requirement to keep the body alive, healthy, fit, and able to perform everyday activities.

Improper intake of food is helping to cause a worldwide pandemic of obesity. Yes,food is making some healty, but it is killing even more. The Introduction Section tells much about the eleven natural products we recommend to lose weight and improve health. These proper information about these NAPS should always be at hand. When you plan your meals, take care in purchasing and consume foods that are healthy, certain illnesses can be prevented. As for the case of obesity, it can be treated through fat burning and weight losing.

The TrimShakes are nutritious meal replacements and should not be consumed along with another regular meal. That will defeat the purpose of using NAPS. At the end of this chapter is an example of a meal made of TrimShake.

Nutritional Wellbeing

According to the Surgeon, Generally, 70 percent of our health status is determined by the lifestyle choices we make—what we eat, drink, whether we smoke, exercise, and even how we love.

Our overall health is determined by our nutritional intake. We should pay careful attention to our food selection process. If you are vegan or vegetarian, you must pay close attention to incorporate a variety of foods for balanced nutrition. The Vegetarian TrimShakes are healthy if you would like to lose weight using the V TrimShake.

Again, to begin, I recommend that you ask God's guidance. Where He leads, He feeds. Just do it! Making the adjustment might take weeks or even months but you must make a good plan and stick-to-it. In the end, it will be worth it.

Trying out different foods or places to eat may cost a little more at first so plan on having a little more money on hand.

The beauty about using NAPS is; you can use more and do not gain extra weight. If you are overweight or obese, you will lose weight instead and keep it off.

Try not to skip meals. It is a great idea to start with a big breakfast, followed by a medium lunch and then a smaller meal for supper.

You may have to develop strong will power to start because support from most people around you may not be positive at first. The interesting thing is, most overweight or obese individual, would love to start a weight management project like you are about to, yet they are the same one who will be first to discourage you. Do not be discouraged by negatives, avoid all and speak workds of encouragement into your own situation. Remember: You become what you think.

SOME DIETARY GUIDELINES FROM THE US GOVERNMENT

If governments are spending trillions of dollars to fix the current healthcare problems our food choices are causing, then surely, they have the right to tell us how and what to eat everyday. The U.S. Departments of Agriculture, Health and Human Services has such programs. "Let's eat for the health of it! Start by choosing one or more tips to help you...

Build a Healthy Plate

Before you eat, think about what goes on your plate or in your cup or bowl. Foods like vegetables, fruits, whole grains, low-fat dairy products, and lean protein foods contain the nutrients you need without too many calories. Try some of these options.

- Make half your plate fruits and vegetables.
- Switch to skim or 1% milk (for meat eaters) for vegans use soy, rice or almond milk substitute
- Make at least half your grains whole.
- Vary your protein food choices.
- Keep your food safe to eat - learn more at www.FoodSafety.gov.
- Cut back on foods high in solid fats, added sugars, and salt

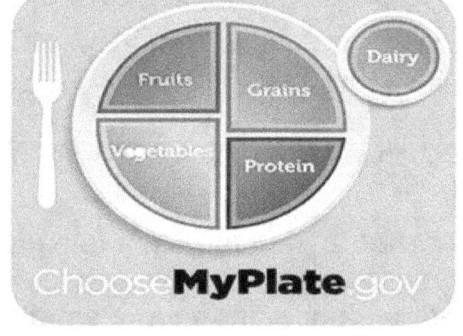

Many people eat foods with too much solid fats, added sugars, and salt (sodium).

Added sugars and fats load foods with extra calories you don't need. Too much sodium may increase your blood pressure. Therefore, remember to:

- Choose foods and drinks with little or no added sugars.
- Look out for salt (sodium) in foods you buy - it all adds up.
- Eat fewer foods that are high in solid fats.

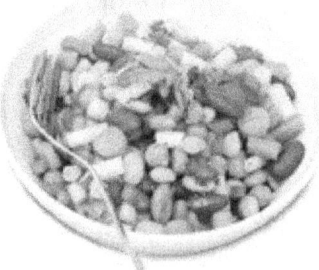

Eat the Right Amount of Calories for You

Everyone has a personal calorie limit. Staying within yours can help you get to or maintain a healthy weight. People who are successful at managing their weight have found ways to keep track of how much they eat in a day, even if they don't count every calorie.

- Enjoy your food, but eat less.
- Cook more often at home, where you are in control of what's in your food and on your plate.
- When eating out, choose lower calorie menu options with reduced fats, salt and sugar.
- Write down what you eat to keep track of how much you eat daily (this is a better way to track intake).
- (Your government says: If you drink alcoholic beverages, do so sensibly - limit to 'one' drink a day for women or to 'two' drinks a day for men.); the bible said: a little wine is good for the stomach's sake…

Be Physically Active Your Way

Pick activities that you like and start by doing what you can, at least 10 minutes at a time. Every bit adds up, and the health benefits increase as you spend more time being active.

Note to parents: What you eat and drink and your level of physical activity are important for your own health, and also for your children's health. You are your children's most important role model. Your children pay attention to what you do more than what you say.

You can do a lot to help your children develop healthy habits for life by providing and eating healthy meals and snacks. For example, don't just tell your children to eat their vegetables - show them that you eat and enjoy vegetables every day. ”

The U.S. Departments of Agriculture and Health and Human Services

CONCLUSION:

How to eat healthy to lose weight everyday, means five little things that must be mastered and they are:

1. **Behavioral Changes** in: Activities, of the mind, body, diet, nutrition, finance
2. **Exercises**: aerobics and anaerobics frequently
3. **Plan, Purchase and Prepare NAPS** products
4. **Attitude Change**: Speak words of positive affirmations into your life
5. **Nutrition: Natural and Healthy. Eat more foods as grown**, less processed foods.

SOME BENEFITS OF EATING HEALTHY

There are thousands of individuals today who desire to lose weight for many reasons such as:

- To stop, prevent or reverse lifestyle diseases.
- It is now reported that "7 out of 10 deaths are now due to cardiovascular disease and cancer".
- 70% of all the deaths are due to heart disease and stroke, and cancer."

As one research pointed out, "this epidemic was never a problem until the emergence of our commercial and scientific advancement because in these now wealthy countries the people once grew their foods and most were too poor to purchase or store meats for everyday consumption but now enters modernization... "

The wealthy have mixed up the entire process. Instead of eating the natural foods as grown to support our bodies, we feed the grains and vegetable to the animals. We then kill these animals, seasoned them with over processed sauces, salt and spices so we can eat their fatty meats. These meats are high in cholesterol and even diseases that clog up our arteries but we forced it all down and even have to at times, washed them into our stomachs with sweet juices.

Our bodies get so tired and listless trying hard to digest these heavy meals that we have to sit down to rest and wait on our over worked heart as it pants for breath. After a time, the heart is the first to go and has now become the greatest cause for our death. We reap the benefits of these fatty meals: overweight, obesity, heart disease, diabetes, hypertension, high cholesterol, triglycerides, and much more...

Some Benefits of Healthy Diet Change

The Coronary Health Improvement Program Newsletter said it best in Lifeline Health Letter, Special Diet Issue. With healthy diet change, we experience:-

- "Blood cholesterol levels come down 15 – 20%, and "elevated cholesterol is the indispensable prerequisite for arterial narrowing writes Dr. Hans Diehl, Dietary Expert,
- Blood pressure and blood sugar levels drop consistently,
- Excess weight drops consistently 6 – 8 lbs. in 4 weeks,
- Depression lifts which lowers the medication requirements,
- Many patients lose their angina pains,
- More than 50% of cancers in Western society are directly related to over nutrition, particularly the high intake of fat.
- Fat-influenced high estrogen levels may hasten the onset of puberty, which increases the risk of breast cancer. Vegetarians have lower levels of blood estrogens. This lowers the risk of breast cancer.
- Diets high in fat and low in fiber promote colon cancer. Diet low in fat and high in fiber protect against it. Fruits and vegetables reduce cancer risk."
- "With a very low fat high fiber diet, 50 – 75% of type 2 diabetics could normalize their blood sugar and get off insulin within weeks." James Anderson MD. The Pritikin Longevity Center and the Diabetes Clinic

Nutritional Information

Nutrition plays a great role in one's health. If you change your diet and eat more natural foods as grown, in moderation, you will begin to lose weight. Continue to incorporate these healthy habits daily and you will not only lose weight but keep the weight off. Let us take some time to familiarize ourselves how healthy eating works. Let us now discuss the different nutrition needed by the body to maintain healthy living and keep our weight at a healthy level.

Carbohydrates

Carbohydrate-rich foods are the primary source of energy needed by the body to perform different daiy chores. Our body breaks down carbohydrates (or carbs) into fuel for use by the cells and muscles – that is why eating a moderate amount of carbohydrates is necessary for most people.

There are two types of carbs: sugars and starches.

1. **Sugars are simple carbohydrates** that can be easily digested by our body, while
2. **Starches are complex carbohydrates** that take longer to be digested.

Many carbohydrate-rich foods are loaded with other nutrients. Fruits and vegetables are not only great carbohydrate sources; they're also excellent suppliers of vitamins A and C and many other vitamins, minerals and fiber. Most dairy products are also great sources of carbohydrates.

Sugar-rich foods: Cake, soda, candy, jellies, and fruits

Starch-rich foods: Breads, grains, pasta, tortillas, noodles, fruits and vegetables

Other carbohydrates-rich food: Fruits and vegetables, and most dairy products

Protein

Along with carbohydrates, our body needs protein – a nutrient made up of essential and non-essential amino acids – for good health. The human body manufactures 13 non-essential amino acids, which are not available from food. For the body to process protein properly, the foods that we eat must contain the 9 essential amino acids that are available only from dietary sources.

Our body is not capable of making these amino acids on its own, so it's critical that you eat foods containing these compounds. The nine essential amino acids are:

- Histidine
- Leucine
- Methionine
- Threonine
- Valine

Isoleucine
Lysine
Phenylalanine
Tryptophan

Where to Find Essential Amino Acids

Individuals should try to get each of the nine essential amino acids in their diet each day.

These amino acids can be found in a variety of different foods which contain protein. The

following is a list of the best sources for the nine essential amino acids:

1. **Histidine**: Histidine is found in the highest concentration in various types of game meat. Deer, boar and antelope are each a top source of histidine. You can get histidine from fish like cod, pike, haddock and tuna. Other sources of histidine include chicken, turkey and kidney beans.

2. **Isoleucine**: If you want to get isoleucine in your diet, your best option is to eat egg whites, which contain by far the most of this amino acid per serving. Turkey is your next best option, following by soy, chicken, and lamb. Many types of fish also contain isoleucine, including pike, roughy, cod and tuna.

3. **Leucine:** Leucine can be found in some interesting foods, including soy, seaweed and elk. However, egg whites are also an excellent source of this amino acid, as is chicken. Tuna is another great option if you are looking for ways to add leucine to your diet.

4. **Lysine**: Lysine is found in the highest concentration in chicken breast meat and turkey breast meat. However, fish is your next best option, with sunfish, tuna, cod, all being excellent sources of lysine as well. Though not as high in concentration, watercress, seaweed and parsley also contain significant amounts of lysine.

5. **Methionine**: As with many other essential amino acids, egg whites are the best source for methionine. However, fish like roughy, pike and tuna aren't far behind. You can also eat meats like turkey and chicken to get this amino acid in your diet.

6. **Phenylalanine**: Meat is the way to go for phenylalanine, which is found in the highest concentration in beef, turkey, veal and lamb. Salmon is also a solid source of this amino acid, however, as are various flours, such as cottonseed flour and sesame flour.

7. **Threonine**: Threonine marks a refreshing break from meats and fish since the top source of this amino acid are raw watercress and spinach. However, you can still get this compound from, turkey or tilapia if you so choose. Egg whites and soy are also

significant sources of threonine.

8. **Tryptophan**: Though it is commonly associated with turkey, especially at Thanksgiving. Other top sources for this amino acid include seaweed, soy, egg whites and spinach.

9. **Valine**: Once again, egg whites come in first when it comes to getting valine in your diet. However, watercress, spinach, seaweed, turkey are also great options for this amino acid.

Protein helps to maintain and replace the tissues in the body. It is found in almost every living cell and fluid. Our muscles, organs and many of our hormones are made up of protein. It is also used in the manufacture of hemoglobin, the red blood cells that carry oxygen to our body. Protein is also used to produce antibodies that fight infections and diseases. Both children and adults need plenty of protein to grow and develop.

There are two kinds of proteins. They are:

1. **Complete protein** – which supplies enough essential amino acids such as Meat, eggs and dairy products – or
2. **Incomplete proteins** – which lacks adequate essential amino acids such as Vegetables, beans and other plant products.

Protein-rich foods: Beef, poultry, lamb; fish and shellfish; dairy products, including cottage cheese, cheese, yogurt and milk; eggs, egg whites or egg substitutes; dry beans, peas, oats and legumes; tofu and soy products; nuts and seeds

Vitamins

Vitamins are organic compounds that help maintain normal body functions, such as reproduction, growth and cell repair. Our body cannot produce vitamins, so we need to obtain them from other sources. Most of the vitamins we need come from the food we eat, except for two: vitamin D, which the body acquires when exposed to sunlight, and vitamin K, which is made by the bacteria in our intestines. In addition to their presence in natural foods, vitamins can also be manufactured synthetically. Vitamin supplements may be available in tablet, capsules, or liquid form. These include:

- **Vitamin A** – affects the formation and maintenance of skin, mucus membranes, bones and teeth, vision, and reproduction. Vitamin A is found in milk, butter, cheese, egg yolk, liver, and fish-liver oil.

- **Vitamin B Complex** – are fragile, water-soluble substances, several of which are particularly important to carbohydrate metabolism. It is composed by vitamin B_1 (thiamine), vitamin B_2 (riboflavin), vitamin B_3 (niacin), vitamin B_6 (pyridoxine), vitamin B_{12} (cobalamin), folic acid, pantothenic acid, and biotin.

- **Vitamin C (Ascorbic acid)** – important in the formation and maintenance of collagen, the protein that supports many body structures and plays a major role in the formation of bones and teeth. Sources of vitamin C include citrus fruits, fresh strawberries, cantaloupe, pineapple, and guava. Good vegetable sources are broccoli, Brussels sprouts, tomatoes, spinach, kale, green peppers, cabbage, and turnips.

- **Vitamin D** – necessary for normal bone formation and for retention of calcium and phosphorus in the body. Also called the sunshine vitamin, vitamin D is obtained from egg yolk, liver, tuna, and vitamin-D fortified milk.

- **Vitamin E** – plays some role in forming red blood cells and muscle and other tissues and in preventing the oxidation of vitamin A and fats. It is found in vegetable oils, wheat germ, liver, and leafy green vegetables.

- **Vitamin K** – necessary mainly for the coagulation of blood. The richest sources of vitamin K are alfalfa and fish livers, which are used in making concentrated preparations of this vitamin. Dietary sources include all leafy green vegetables, egg yolks, soybean oil, and liver.

  All THE NAPS products has the correct amounts of nutrients your body needs.

Minerals

Minerals are small amounts of metallic elements that are vital for the healthy growth of teeth and bones. They also help in cellular activities such as enzyme action, muscle contraction, nerve reaction, and blood clotting. Mineral nutrients are classified as major elements (calcium, chlorine, magnesium, phosphorus, potassium, sodium, and sulfur) and trace elements (chromium, copper, fluoride, iodine, iron, selenium, and zinc).

How Much Fat To Consume?

Do not give in to this very common misconception in the area of food and nutrition that fat is always bad for health. We have already mentioned earlier that when more calories are eaten than the body needs, the body stores those additional calories as fat, causing subsequent overweight and obesity. That's only when fat becomes unwanted.

Fat is the body's major energy storage system. When the energy from the food we eat and drink can't be used by our body, the body turns it into fat for later use. The body uses fat from foods for energy, to cushion organs and bones, and to make hormones and regulate blood pressure. Some fat is also necessary to maintain healthy skin, hair and nails. Thus, one should not eliminate all fat from the diet. But, remember that too much fat can lead to many health problems such as heart disease, obesity, diabetes and more.

From above, we can entail that not all fats are created equal. There are the saturated fats – the unhealthy ones – and the unsaturated fats – the good and healthy ones.

Saturated Fat: Unhealthy Fats

Saturated fats, which are generally solid at room temperature, are the least healthy and tend to increase the level of cholesterol in our blood. Foods that contain saturated fat include butter, cheese, margarine, shortening, tropical oils such as coconut and palm oil, and the fats in meat and poultry skin. Consumption of these oils and foods should be limited. Otherwise, they may bring serious health diseases.

Unsaturated Fat: Healthy Ones

Unsaturated fats reduce blood cholesterol when they replace saturated fats in the diet. There are two types of unsaturated fat: monounsaturated fat and polyunsaturated fat. **Monounsaturated fats** have been shown to raise the level of HDL – the 'good' cholesterol that protects against heart attacks – in the blood, so in moderation they can be part of a healthy diet. This is why they are known as the good fats; although, consumption of these should also be given attention. Olive and canola oils, peanut butter and nuts are particularly high in monounsaturated fats.

Weight Loss Diets

Losing weight means losing body fat. And losing body fat means any of two ways: limiting the intake of high-fat foods or consuming fat-burning foods. Either of these ways will not only improve one's metabolism, but it will also allow him more food for his calorie expenditure because fats have more than twice the calories per gram as proteins (which contain 4 calories per gram) and carbohydrates.

Low-Fat Diet

This is the ideal diet for prevention of overweight or obesity. A low-fat diet involves intake of food with little fat calories instead of those with high fat calories. This is advisable for those who still do not suffer from obesity and want to avoid go through it. Most parents refer to this type of diet for their children due to fear that they might grow obese. Below is a diet suggestion for general good health or for dietary treatment. Foods are categorize according to low-fat (allowed to consume) and high-fat (prohibited to consume):

Fat-Burning Diet

Fat-burning diet is about burning unwanted fat calories that is stored in the body. Certain foods and eating habits can be used to accelerate fat-burning, either directly promoting the meltdown of the body's stored fats, or indirectly by modifying our energy use. These foods include:

☐ **Protein-Rich Foods** – significantly increase the metabolic rate (the pace at which we use food fuel), creating heat and burning many more calories than carbohydrates or fat.

<u>Fat-Burner Protein Foods</u>

☐ **Lean Meat:** Beef, lamb, veal, add your choice

☐ **Poultry:** Chicken, turkey, add your choice here

☐ **Fish:** Cod, haddock, sole, whiting, trout, salmon, add your choice

☐ **Cheese:** Mainly low-fat cottage cheese and low-fat fromage frais. Use reduced-fat versions of hard cheeses, such as Cheddar, in moderation

☐ **Eggs**

☐ **Soya products**

☐ **Negative Calorie Foods** – use up more calories to break down, digest, and assimilate them than they supply. Eating mainly negative calorie foods is said to reduce weight three times faster than fasting and to reduce body weight by an average of 0.5 kg (1 lb) a day

<u>Negative-Calorie Foods</u>

Vegetables: Asparagus, aubergine (eggplant), beetroot, broccoli, Brussels sprouts, cabbage, carrots, cauliflower, celeriac, celery, chicory, Chinese cabbage (pak choi, bok choi), cress, dandelion leaves, endive, fennel, globe artichokes, green beans, leeks, lettuce, mangetouts (snow peas), mooli (daikon or Japanese radish), mushrooms, okra (ladies' fingers), onions, radishes, seaweed, spinach, squash, swede, tomatoes, turnips hazelnuts, macademias, peanuts, pine nuts, pistachios, walnuts

Fruits: Apples, apricots, bananas, blackberries, blackcurrants, blueberries, boysenberries, cherries, clementines, cranberries, damsons, figs, gooseberries, grapefruit, grapes, greengages, guavas, kiwi fruit, kumquat, loquat, lychees, mandarins, mangos, medlars, melons, mulberries, nectarines, oranges, papaya, peaches, pears, persimmons, pineaaple, plums, pomegranate, prickly pear, raspberries, redcurrants, satmusas, star fruit, strawberries, whitecurrants

Nuts: Almonds, Barcelona nuts, Brazil nuts, chestnuts, coconuts, filberts

☐ **Low-GI (Glycaemic Index) Carbohydrate Foods** – help us to burn up the food at our disposal rather than storing it as fat

Low-GI Carbohydrate Foods

☐ **Breads:** Multigrain breads (white and brown), heavy fruit breads

☐ **Grains and Breakfast Cereals:** Brown rice, wild rice, other whole grains,

☐ tabbouleh, pearl barley, whole wheat pasta, oats, porridge,

☐ unsweetened muesli, high-fiber wheat bran cereal

☐ **Vegetables:** Sweet potato, okra mushrooms, legumes (peas, beans),

☐ broccoli, artichokes

☐ **Fruits:** Apples, pears, oranges, mandarins, grapefruit, bananas

☐ **Other:** Honey, jam, Soya milk and its products

SIMPLE RECIPES

Cucumber Avocado Open-faced Sandwiches

Ingredients:

1 loaf thinly sliced artisan multigrain bread
1-2 avocados
1 wedge semi-soft cheese with herbs (we used Fromage d'Affinois), room temperature
1 British cucumber
1 small package microgreens
1 drop Thyme essential oil
Salt and pepper, to taste

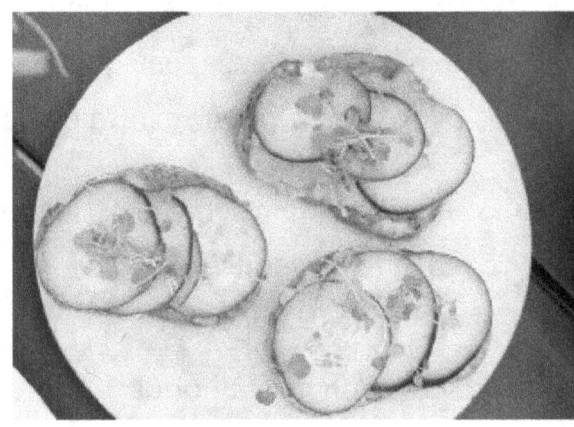

Directions:

1. Slice cucumber, pat to dry. Set aside. Lay out bread slices. Mash avocados, adding 1 drop of Thyme essential oil plus salt and pepper to taste.
2. Spread bread slices with cheese, then avocado mixture. Place cucumber slices on top and sprinkle with more salt and pepper. Add a flourish of microgreens and serve immediately

Green Machine Smoothie with Slim & Sassy TrimShake

Servings: 1   **Prep Time: 3 min.**
      Difficulty: Easy

Ingredients:

1 scoop vanilla TrimShake
1 cup unsweetened original almond milk
1 drop Wild Orange essential oil
1 cup frozen fruit of your choice
1/3 cup vanilla yogurt
1 tablespoon chia seeds
2–3 cups raw spinach

Instructions: Blend until Smooth

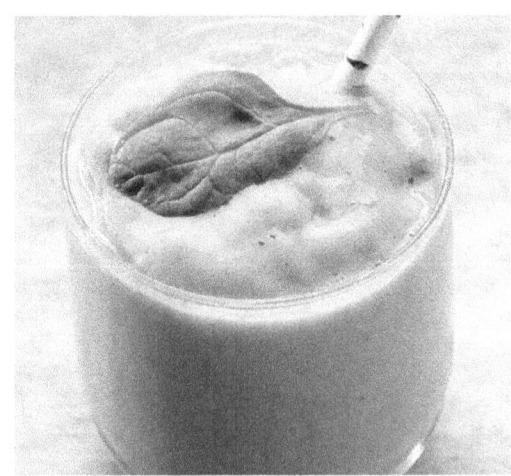

Figure 12 Vanilla TrimShake

BONUS # 4

The Proper Exercises To Lose Weight

It is an accepted fact that exercise is an important part of any successful weight loss plan. Every muscle you have can burn calories, so the more you work them, the more calories you burn. The Natural Appetite-control Products and Supplements are great especially when combined with exercises to lose weight. Yes, diet is important but don't just depend on dieting. Do some exercises to achieve that weight you have always dreamed about but most importantly to guard against diseases, to look and feel great.

Deep Breathing

Although deep breathing alone can not eliminate those excess fats hanging by your belly or legs, it will make you calmer, stress free and will give you increased energy to use throughout the day. Any new positive habits cultivated will help to encourage you on.

When to do Deep breathing

Do deep breathing exercises upon waking in the morning, before going to sleep at night, and at least once during the day.

How to do Deep Breathing

Stand easily, or lie down if you happen to be on bed – whichever's more comfortable and convenient for you. Take a deep breath **slowly** over a count of 5 seconds. Fill your lungs with fresh air as full as possible. Hold your breath for 20 seconds or for as long as you can without straining yourself, and then breathe out again very slowly to a count of 10. Repeat a total of 15 times.

Walking

Walking is great exercise to lose weight. Moreover, it does not require any expertise or equipment and you can do it free anytime you feel like it. However, to be beneficial, you should do it frequently.

When to Walk

Make walking a daily habit or at least 3-5 times a week depending on your schedule.

How to Walk

Before you start walking, do some warm up stretching exercises. Stretch only as far as you feel comfortable so as not to make any fractures. Start with a modest goal, like 15 to 20 minutes at a leisurely pace. Gradually extend the duration and the speed. Walk up one or two gentle slopes. Your walk should be comprised of three segments: warm-up, exercise pace and cool-down.

Walking –But Doing it Right

- Walk with your chin up and your shoulders held slightly back.

- The heel of your foot should touch the ground first. Roll your weight forward.

- Swing your arms as you walk.

- To avoid stiff or sore muscles or joints, start gradually. Over several weeks, begin walking faster, going further, and walking for longer periods of time.

- Walk on soft ground.

- Quench yourself – drink 8-10 ounces of water for every 20 minutes of the activity. This recommendation may not be for everyone. If you are sick, **check with your healthcare provider first before start exercising or drinking too much water**.

Benefits of Walking

Exercise has many benefits and walking is a great exercise. The more you walk, the better you will feel. Plus, walking also uses more calories; thus, burning more fats. Its benefits include giving you more energy, making you feel good, helping you to relax, reducing stress, helping you sleep better, toning your muscles, helping control your appetite, and increasing the number of calories your body uses.

To lose weight, it's more important to walk for time than speed. Walking at a moderate pace yields longer workouts with less soreness – leading to more miles and more calories spent on a regular basis. This is a great habit to develop because the benefits are long term.

Aerobic Exercises

The word *aerobic* literally means "with oxygen" or "in the presence of oxygen." Aerobic exercise is any activity that uses large muscle groups, can be maintained continuously for a long period of time and is rhythmic in nature.

Aerobic exercises utilize oxygen as the major fuel for sustaining activity for relatively long periods. Over all, aerobic exercises are those activities that require large muscle work outs, elevate the heart rate to between 60 percent and 80 percent of maximal heart rate, are continuous in nature, and are of 15 to 60 minutes in duration. An aerobically fit individual can work longer, more vigorously and achieve a quicker recovery at the end of the aerobic session.

Types of Aerobic Exercises

Aerobic exercises fall in two categories:

a. **Low to Moderate-Impact Exercises** – These include walking, swimming, stair climbing, step classes, rowing, and cross-country skiing. Nearly anyone in reasonable health can engage in some low - to moderate-impact exercise. Brisk walking burns as many calories as jogging for the same distance and poses less risk for injury to muscle and bone.

b. **High-Impact Exercises** – Activities that belong to this group include running, dance exercise, tennis, racquetball, and squash. High-impact exercises should be performed only every alternate day. People who are overweight, obese, elderly, out of condition, or have an injury or other medical problem should do them even less frequently.

Some Aerobic Exercises

1. Walking

Walking is a popular form of exercise because it requires little in terms of equipment or facilities. Walking an extra 20 minutes each day will burn off 7 pounds of body fat per year. Longer, moderately-paced daily walks are best for losing weight.

2. Jogging/Running

When jogging or running, an individual is able to cover greater distances in a shorter period of time. Therefore, greater numbers of calories can be burned.

3. Choreographed Aerobic Exercise

Choreographed aerobic dance is a very popular form of exercise throughout the world. Aerobic dance helps in toning up the muscles of the body.

4. Step Aerobics

Step aerobics involves the use of a step or bench typically about one foot wide and three feet long and about six inches high. Instructors use many moves that require participants to step up and down from the platform. This way, the activity will not be boring and tiring, but will be lively and motivating.

5. Water Aerobics

Water aerobics involves a variety of movements from both swimming and land aerobics to develop vigorous routines that are aerobic in nature. It utilizes the resistance to movement that water creates to elevate heart rates. It helps in losing weight.

6. Swimming

Swimming is a very popular form of exercise. Due to the resistance of water, the amount of energy required to swim a certain distance is greater than that needed to run or walk the same distance. That is why, swimming burns more calories than running.

7. Stationary Cycling/Bicycling

Stationary cycling or bicycling is excellent forms of aerobic exercise when done continuously. Just like swimming, cycling is a non weight bearing activity that builds muscular endurance and strength which improved flexibility of selected muscles of the legs and thighs. To avoid boredom, add your favorite music. I do this exercise regularly with great results.

8. Jumping Rope

Jumping rope can be a great aerobic workout as long as it is performed at a slow to moderate pace and is done continuously for a relatively long period of time (15 minutes).

The key to effective weight loss is through use of a healthy exercise program which is performed on a regular basis while following a healthy eating and the 30-day lose weight nutritional plan. Aerobic exercise is good to lose weight because it uses more calories than other activities and helps raise ones metabolic rate which helps the body burn calories at a faster rate. It is an effective way to lose fat only if you are motivated enough to workout frequently. Aerobics only burn fat during the workout so if you want encouraging results you need to be able to exercise frequently and for longer periods.

Cardiovascular Exercises

This form of exercise is one of the best ways to burn a lot of calories while losing extra body fat and giving the metabolism a big boost. Cardio exercises are those that raise your heart rate to 65-90% of your maximum heart rate.

Cardiovascular fitness is considered to be the most important area of physical fitness. Cardiovascular fitness is based on maximizing oxygen intake. This is best achieved through physical activity involving large muscle groups over prolonged period of time. These activities are rhythmic and aerobic in nature such as walking, running, hiking, stair climbing, swimming, cycling, rowing, dancing, skating, cross country skiing, rope jumping, and many more.

When to do Cardiovascular Exercises

Traditionally, the best time to do cardio exercises to gain the for maximum fat loss is early in the morning before you eat anything. After you've been asleep for 6-8 hours, the level of sugar (glucose) in your blood is very low and your body will use stored fat more easily as an alternative energy source. Now, if you are a diabetic, please check your glucose levels before starting any exercise and this is a must anytime of the day.

Benefits of Cardiovascular Exercises

- Increases calorie and fat burn

- To lose weight

- Reduces the risk of heart disease

- Increased lung capacity

- Reduced blood pressure

- Prevents diabetes

- Increase metabolism (see BMR)

- Strengthens the cardiovascular system

- Strengthens the immune system

- Lowers stress levels

Weight Training

Some authorities claim that this is the best fat-burning exercise on the grounds since the metabolism continues to burn at an increased rate for 24 hours after a 60-minute workout. However, weight training leads to development of greater lean muscle mass with its ability to utilize calories more efficiently.

Weight training also firms and tones the body, while combating any muscular wastage that can result from prolonged dieting. Together with aerobic exercise or increased regular exercise, helps to boost the body's metabolism when the calorie intake is reduced.

Weight training is best done at your local gym since they have complete equipment. Plus, there are programs where you can enroll with an instructor to guide you with the right exercises, number of repetitions, and duration of each activity. In such places, they will monitor your weight loss and guarantee your safety. On the other hand, if you can afford to buy the right equipments for weight training and work out, then you could do the activity right inside your home.

It is importnt that you educate yourself well before beginning your weight training program at home to avoid injury to yourself. My husband watches Youtube videos before he started his weight training at home and he is doing very well. He has lost over 30 pounds and toned up. It is more convenient for him to work out at home and this may be the same for you. In that way, you can exercise whenever you want.

Exercise Tools and Equipments

These exercise tools and equipments are related to weight training and work out since they can not be done without these things, unlike the previous four exercises which need only your body, energy, and presence of mind. Advanced exercise machines include electronic devices that measure your weight before and after you do the exercise, the amount of calories you burned, time elapsed, and other useful information.

Treadmill

A treadmill is an exercise device consisting of an endless belt on which an individual can walk or jog without changing place .It is supported by a sturdy deck driven either by an electric motor or by the use. It generally has some shock absorption system, usually rubber cushioning, to minimize stress on the joints.

Using a treadmill will speed up your metabolic rate and allow your body to absorb and utilize a greater quantity of nutrients that you consume. It will also stabilize your insulin levels and blood sugar as well as increase your energy level.

Using a treadmill to lose weight, you need to exercise on a daily basis. A treadmill helps you burn more calories by increasing your exercise frequency. It gives you a LOT of workout versatility. You can start with a slow walk and then speed it up as your body gets into better shape. By using the large muscles of the legs, a treadmill helps you burn major fat calories.

Elliptical Trainer

Elliptical trainers are exercise machines, which combine the natural stride of a treadmill and the simplicity of a stair climber. On an Elliptical trainer, you position yourself comfortably in an upright position while holding onto the machine's handrails and striding in either a forward or reverse motion.

The elliptical trainer burns more calories than either the treadmill or the exercise bike. With an elliptical cross trainer, you get the benefits of weight bearing exercises such as jogging without the wear and tear on your joints. It provides a great cardio workout that pumps you heart to the max without the strain and stress on your joints. It uses all of the muscles of the lower leg. Therefore, you will strengthen and build your lower legs. This is an ideal workout for the overweight or obese individual who do not want to jog.

Exercise Bikes

There are two types of exercise bikes you can use, upright bikes and recumbent bikes. Upright bikes simulate the action of a real bike except you do not go anywhere. Recumbent bikes on the other hand, have bucket seats which have the pedals out in front of you.

Exercise bikes are great for cardiovascular fitness and toning or building your thighs. The recumbent bikes are especially good for toning your butt. Being stationary, you can enjoy your favorite magazine or TV program while working out.

For overweight or obese people, the recumbent bike offers bucket seats which can be more comfortable than traditional uprights. This type of bike is more ergonomically correct than a traditional upright exercise bike and an effective way to improve aerobic capacity, as well as burn fat. It offers more back support and may be a little more comfortable to those people with lower back pain.

Rowers

There are two types of rowing machines. A hydraulic machine uses a piston to provide the resistance. With a cable-driven machine, your pull spins a flywheel which produces a smooth action similar to rowing on water. The smoothness of the flywheel creates little strain on the back. **Important:** If handles are not adjusted properly for height differences, hydraulic rowers can create back strain.

Rowing machines provide a whole-body aerobic workout: arms, shoulders, back, abdomen, legs, heart and lungs. It also builds muscle strength and endurance in addition to the aerobic benefits. It improves your whole cardiovascular system with a low impact workout. Other benefits include improved flexibility and muscle strengthening in the arms, abdomen, and back. On the other hand, its disadvantage includes not causing the pounding on the legs and knees that running does.

Steppers

Steppers are available as simple step-bench or as computerized stair steppers. It tones the buttocks, thighs and hips. These are those areas that have a tendency to "balloon" from too many calories and not enough exercise. Stair stepper work outs are calorie burners that rank as one of the best cardiovascular exercises for people of all ages and fitness levels.

WHAT STOPS YOU FROM EXERCISING?

IF YOU ARE HAVING PAIN DURING OR AFTER EXERCISE, USE DEEP BLUE SOOTHING BLEND

Deep Blue® Soothing Blend

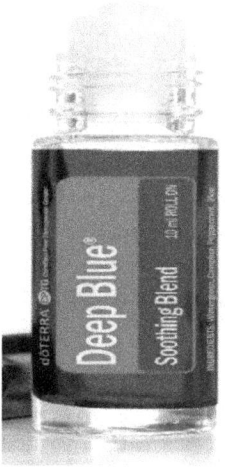

Formulated to soothe and cool, doTERRA Deep Blue serves as an enriching blend of oils perfect for a massage after a long day or an intense workout.

Part Number: 31050001   Size: 5 mL
Wholesale: $32.00   Retail: $42.67   PV: 32

Figure 13 Deep Blue Soothing Blend

Description

doTERRA Deep Blue is perfect for a soothing massage after a long day of work. Wintergreen, Camphor, Peppermint, Ylang-Ylang, Helichrysum, Blue Tansy, Blue Chamomile, and Osmanthus work together to soothe and cool. After long hours on the computer, try rubbing Deep Blue proprietary blend on your fingers, wrists, shoulders, and neck. A few drops of Deep Blue Soothing Blend diluted in Fractionated Coconut Oil can be part of a cooling and comforting massage.

Uses

- Apply on feet and knees before and after exercise.
- Massage Deep Blue with a few drops of carrier oil onto growing kids' legs before bedtime.
- Rub Deep Blue on lower back muscles after a day of heavy lifting at work or during a move.

Directions for Use

Topical use: Apply to desired area. Dilute with dōTERRA Fractionated Coconut Oil to minimize any skin sensitivity.

Cautions

Possible skin sensitivity. Keep out of reach of children. If you are pregnant, nursing, or under a doctor's care, consult your physician. Avoid contact with eyes, inner ears, and sensitive areas.

Primary Benefits

- Soothing and cooling oil blend, Comforting part of a massage

All Natural Ingredients

Wintergreen, Camphor, Peppermint, Ylang-Ylang, Helichrysum, Blue Tansy, Blue Chamomile, and Osmanthus

Aromatic Description: Minty, camphoraceous

Click to Buy Now: Deep Blue® Soothing Blend or Copy and Paste in Browser: http://bit.ly/2lEZ8V5

Description

dōTERRA Deep Blue Rub is a rich, topical cream infused with the Deep Blue Soothing Blend of CPTG Certified Pure Therapeutic Grade essential oils. Formulated with a proprietary blend of natural plant extracts and other powerful ingredients, Deep Blue Rub provides a comforting sensation of cooling and warmth to problem areas. With close to 5 mL of dōTERRA's top-selling Deep Blue essential oil blend of Wintergreen, Camphor, Peppermint, Ylang-Ylang, Helichrysum, Blue Tansy, Blue Chamomile, and Osmanthus, Deep Blue Rub is an essential addition to your bathroom cabinet, gym bag, or first aid kit. Deep Blue Rub is blended in a base of moisturizing emollients that leave your skin feeling soft and not greasy. It is the choice of massage therapists and sports practitioners who currently use dōTERRA's Deep Blue proprietary blend in their practice.

Uses

Massage lotion into affected areas. For a more intensive treatment, apply Deep Blue Soothing Blend on the skin prior to lotion application.

Cautions

For external use, only. Avoid contact with eyes. Do not use on wounds or damaged skin. Do not bandage tightly after application or use with a heating pad. Keep out of reach of children to avoid accidental ingestion. If swallowed, get medical help or contact a Poison Control Center immediately.

Deep Blue is now available in a 10ml roll-on

Deep Blue® Rub

dōTERRA Deep Blue Rub is a topical cream formulated with Deep Blue Soothing Blend of CPTG Certified Pure Therapeutic Grade® essential oils, natural plant extracts, and additional helpful ingredients that provides a comforting sensation of cooling and warmth to problem areas.

Primary Benefits

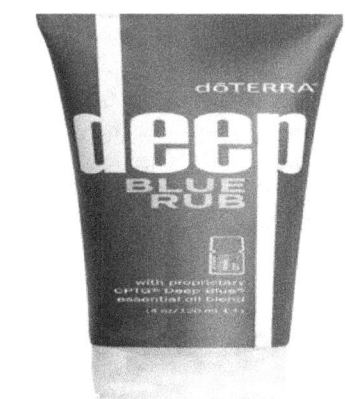

- Formulated with the Deep Blue proprietary blend of essential oils and other powerful ingredients
- Perfect for the athlete in your life, Deep Blue Rub is blended in a base of moisturizing emollients that leaves your skin soft and non-greasy
- Provides a cooling and soothing sensation to targeted areas

Figure 14 Deep Blue® Rub

Click to Buy Now: Deep Blue® Rub
or Copy and Paste in Browser: http://bit.ly/2IEZ8V5

Deep Blue® Rub

dōTERRA Deep Blue Rub is a topical cream formulated with Deep Blue Soothing Blend of CPTG Certified Pure Therapeutic Grade® essential oils, natural plant extracts, and additional helpful ingredients that provides a comforting sensation of cooling and warmth to problem areas.

Part Number: 38900001   Size: 4 fl oz
Wholesale: $29.25   Retail: $39.00   PV: 29.25

Description

dōTERRA Deep Blue Rub is a rich, topical cream infused with the Deep Blue Soothing Blend of CPTG Certified Pure Therapeutic Grade essential oils. Formulated with a proprietary blend of natural plant extracts and other powerful ingredients, Deep Blue Rub provides a comforting sensation of cooling and warmth to problem areas. With close to 5 mL of dōTERRA's top-selling Deep Blue essential oil blend of Wintergreen, Camphor, Peppermint, Ylang-Ylang, Helichrysum, Blue Tansy, Blue Chamomile, and Osmanthus, Deep Blue Rub is an essential addition to your bathroom cabinet, gym bag, or first aid kit. Deep Blue Rub is blended in a base of moisturizing emollients that leave your skin feeling soft and not greasy. It is the choice of massage therapists and sports practitioners who currently use dōTERRA's Deep Blue proprietary blend in their practice.

Uses

Massage lotion into affected areas. For a more intensive treatment, apply Deep Blue Soothing Blend on the skin prior to lotion application.

Cautions

For external use, only. Avoid contact with eyes. Do not use on wounds or damaged skin. Do not bandage tightly after application or use with a heating pad. Keep out of reach of children to avoid accidental ingestion. If swallowed, get medical help or contact a Poison Control Center immediately.

ENCOURAGEMENT TO THE OVERWEIGHT OR OBESE

"If you're experiencing stagnancy in your life, or have

found yourself with little inspiration, minimal confidence,

or greater pessimism, take time to make a change with

dōTERRA Motivate and propel your life in the direction of

creativity and purpose." ONE BOTTLE OF MOTIVATE WILL

HELP CHANGE YOUR LIFE!

USE MOTIVATE ENCOURAGING BLEND ESSENTIAL OIL

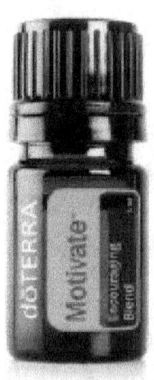

Figure 15 dōTERRA Motivate® Encouraging Blend

dōTERRA Motivate Product Description

dōTERRA Motivate essential oil blend is formulated with mint and citrus essential oils that inspire the senses, allowing you to tear down the demotivating road blacks that stand between you and your potential. Whether you need motivation to clean your room, start training for a race, or pick up your paintbrush again, dōTERRA Motivate blend can support you with the courage and confidence to replace a pessimistic outlook on life with an optimistic one full of possibilities.

Where to Buy dōTERRA Motivate

Something unique to dōTERRA essential oil blends is their composition. All essential oils blends from dōTERRA are made up of CPTG Certified Pure Therapeutic Grade® essential oils. When oils are classified as CPTG®, they have passed the CPTG protocol, which involves a series of rigorous tests that assess the purity, potency, and quality of each batch of essential oils. When you purchase a blend from dōTERRA, you can be confident knowing that the essential oil products you receive are pure and potent, and ready to meet your needs.

The purity and potency of an essential oil is crucial to its effectivity. These qualities are so critical because when essential oils are filled with filler substances and impurities, as many oils on the market are, their quality and effectivity are diminished. However, when oils are pure and potent, they can work properly and effectively to enhance well-being.

dōTERRA Motivate Uses and Benefits

1. Too often, feelings of worthlessness, apprehension, and weakness can cloud thoughts and limit potential. When you feel, these feelings start to weigh on you, use the dōTERRA Motivate blend topically or aromatically for a boost of positive emotion. dōTERRA Motivate oil blend can promote feelings of confidence, courage, and belief and will help you become a more positive and more inspired you.

2. If setbacks and disappointments have you down on yourself or are starting to have a discouraging effect on your emotions, it may be time to regroup and restore you to a more positive outlook. In times like these, use dōTERRA Motivate as an encouraging companion to steer you away from negative emotions. dōTERRA Motivate will help counteract the damaging emotions of doubt, pessimism, and cynicism.

3. In need of a boost of confidence before a performance or speech? Here's a little essential oil tip specifically for those moments. Simply apply dōTERRA Motivate oil blend to a shirt collar or a piece of clothing that is close to the face, and the blend's aroma will give you the self-assurance you need to perform your best.

4. When working on a long paper for school or spending hours on a project, add one or two drops of dōTERRA Motivate blend to the diffuser of your choice and diffuse.

This fresh and minty blend will help you stay motivated and determined so that you can complete your projects.

5. Once you've taken the step to get up and press forward, continue to use the dōTERRA Motivate essential oil blend to encourage and motivate you in your endeavors. If you are a part of sporting events or other competitions, apply dōTERRA Motivate oil to your pulse points before participating. This will give you a positive surge of confidence that will assist you in doing your best.

Chemistry of dōTERRA Motivate

dōTERRA Motivate is formulated with a blend of citrus and mint essential oils such as Yuzu, Clementine, and Peppermint. These oils come together to create a chemical profile that is high in monoterpenes and monoterpene alcohols, which contain uplifting and toning properties. If you would like to learn more about the chemical backgrounds of other aromatherapy oils, visit the dōTERRA Emotional Aromatherapy™ page.

Key Ingredients

- Peppermint Plant
- Coriander Seed
- Yuzu Peel
- Rosemary Leaf

Clementine Peel
Basil Herb
Melissa Leaf
Vanilla Bean Absolute

Cautions

Possible skin sensitivity. Keep out of reach of children. If pregnant or under a doctor's care, consult your physician. Avoid contact with eyes, inner ears, and sensitive areas. Avoid sunlight or UV rays for up to 12 hours after applying product.

Click to Buy Now: Motivate® Encouraging Blend
or Copy and Paste in Browser: http://bit.ly/2IEZ8V5

dōTERRA Motivate® Encouraging Blend

Feelings of confidence and courage will replace negative emotions like guilt and pessimism, with the dōTERRA Motivate Encouraging Blend of mint and citrus essential oils.

Part Number: 31740001   Size: 5 mL
Wholesale: $23.00   Retail: $30.67   PV: 23

- Promotes feelings of confidence, courage, and belief
- Counteracts negative emotions of doubt, pessimism, and cynicism

Description

Are you frustrated at work or have setbacks in life even with your best efforts to improve your confidence? Or has misplaced trust left you cynical more often than your best self should be? Then stop, reset, and restart using your dōTERRA Motivate Encouraging Blend of mint and citrus essential oils. dōTERRA Motivate will help you unleash your creative powers and find the courage that comes from believing in yourself again. Go ahead and raise the bar–you can do it! Features Peppermint Plant, Clementine Peel, Coriander Seed, Basil Herb, Yuzu Peel, Melissa Leaf, Rosemary Leaf, Vanilla Bean.

Uses

- Apply to shirt collar before giving a speech to instill feelings of confidence.
- Diffuse when working on a project at work or school to stay motivated.
- Apply to pulse points before participating in sporting events or other competitions.

Directions for Use

Diffusion: Use one to two drops in the diffuser of your choice.
Topical use: Apply one to two drops to desired area. Dilute with dōTERRA Fractionated Coconut Oil to minimize any skin sensitivity.

Cautions

Possible skin sensitivity. Keep out of reach of children. If pregnant or under a doctor's care, consult your physician. Avoid contact with eyes, inner ears, and sensitive areas. Avoid sunlight or UV rays for up to 12 hours after applying product.

THE LACK OF EXERCISE ALONG WITH OVER EATING LEADS TO OBESITY.

ITS YOUR TURN TO LOSE WEIGHT, MOTIVATE YOURSELF.

Where to Begin? Start at the top—in your head. Before you can lose weight, you must first make the choice to do something about your lifestyle: diet and activity. That decision-making process takes place in the frontal lobe of our brain located in your head. To lose weight starts as a mental process. This involve **planning** how to achieve this. You may need to add, delete or improve some things in your life. New learning takes place in the head, this book has great examples of how to lose weight. Implement some.

Secondly, develop strong belief and trust. You must believe in your ability to stick with the changes until they become a habit that takes over the old ways that led to obesity. Most people cannot do this major shift on their own. That is why so many failed. Others at this junction, called on the Holy Spirit for empowerment to endure. To achieve the proper results, you must exercise wisdom in our choices.

You cannot be lazy about exercising, **purchasing and preparing** your own food. Fast foods are loaded with too much of the wrong ingredients and not enough of good nutrients the body needs for abundant health and functioning. When tempted to give up or give in, seek the Holy Spirit's help. Proverbs 13:4 *"The soul of a lazy man desires, and has nothing; But the soul of the diligent shall be made rich."*

I have done quite a bit of research on how to lose weight and discovered that many authors have avoided this fundamental area of success—faith and trust in God to help with the addiction to sugar, salt, fats and lack of exercising. You must have faith in yourself to fight and stop digging your own grave slowly. You must develop faith in God to help you. There's nothing too hard for the LORD to do. But you must ask His help and ….

Copy Good Leaders

Hebrews 6:12 " *That you do not become sluggish, but imitate those who through faith and patience inherit the promises."* (Promises from God waiting to be claimed by people in need. Ask. Believe. Claim. Do.)

Whatever the reason you are presently overweight or obese, you can get out of it with effort and determination. Never use food or drinks as a substitute for coping with life's challenges or setbacks. Addiction untreated, will lead into further setbacks, lifestyle diseases and poverty.

BONUS # 5

The Proper Lifestyle to Lose Weight: What Is It?

How you live your life affects if you gain or lose weight. You can't expect to lose weight no matter how long you exercise daily if you keep on eating the wrong foods every day. You will get out of life exactly what you have put in. Poor results from poor habits. You will eventually get slim, fit and sassy when you believe in your ability to cut the addiction to sugar, salt, fats and lack of frequent exercising.

Your body needs exercise to maintain itself properly. Start a regular exercise program then plan, purchase and prepare your meals. If you grudge your heart of abundant health and instead behave like a couch-potato in front of the TV set for hours at a time, you will get what the photo got--fried. If your lifestyle is like this, a change is needed. Let us help you kick those unhealthy habits and start getting rid of the 'weights' that so easily beset you.

There are two kinds of weights we are talking about here. They are caused from:

1. Fats that affect the body. It become plaque which clog the arteries. This leads to the number one killer in the USA today, heart attacks.

2. The second weights are our thoughts or emotions that affect the mind. Things Ephesians speak about that keeps us back from excelling to our best potential but instead set us up to grieve the Holy Spirit of God and keep us our of our blessings. We become stiff-necked because of things such as: doubts, fears, anger, bitterness, hatred, malice, spitefulness, selfishness, anxiety, greed,

laziness, wrong habits, wrong choices and more. Paul wrote about them in Ephesians 4: 25 – 31

"Do Not Refuse the Spirit by Whom You Are Helped.

(25) Therefore, putting away lying, "Let each one of you speak truth with his neighbor, for we are members of one another. (26) "Be angry, and do not sin": Do not let the sun go down on your wrath, (27) nor give place to the devil. (28) Let him who stole steal no longer, but rather let him labor, working with his hands what is good, that he may have something to give him who has need. (29) Let no corrupt word proceed out of your mouth, but what is good for necessary edification, that it may impart grace to the hearers. (30) And do not grieve the Holy Spirit of God, by whom you were sealed for the day of redemption. (31) Let all bitterness, wrath, anger, clamor, and evil speaking be put away from you, with all malice." Paul forgot to admonish us to stop procrastination, a #1 thief.

Below are some tips that help to lose weight by burning calories and fats. These simple things that are usually taken for granted will really help you achieve your goal if you stick to it. Making these part of your everyday life will surely make you realize that you should have done those things earlier, but it is never too late to lose weight. Just start.

Good Tips to Lose Weight Everyday

Drink Clear Water

- Drink at least 8 glasses of water everyday if doctor approved. This way, dehydration, which reduces metabolic rate by 2-3%, is avoided. Water itself helps cut down on water retention because it acts as a diuretic. Before meals water can dull the appetite.

- Drink hot water with lemon. Or purchase a bottle of doTERRA'S CPTG lemon oil and use throughout the day in your water.

- Avoid consuming large quantities of fattening liquids, which are so easy to overdo.

- Use the Slim & Sassy Metabolic Blend in your juice. Add it to your water. Sometimes, cravings for food are really thirst in disguise.

Take Natural Appetite-control Products & Supplements - NAPS

- After you purchase your NAPS Metabolic Blend or your New You Kit, use one of the Metabolic Blend . Add drops in your water bottle and drink between meals.

- This will help you cut down on food cravings and the munchies

- Drink the TrimShakes once or twice daily. Followed by a regular meal.

- Do not skip breakfast. Always in-a-hurry-people tend to forget eating early in the morning and ended up eating too much at lunch. Eating breakfast raises metabolic rate by between 10 and 25%. The TrimShakes are great for on the run lifestyle.

- Eat the Metabolic Blend chewing gum between meals to help with chavings.

Do Not Practice Using Crash Diets

- Avoid crash-diets. This lowers metabolic rate, deprives you of essential nutrients.

- Spread your fat over the course of a day. When you are obese, a lot of fat eaten all at once can sharpen the appetite for further fat. Cravings which is addiction.

- Stretch your meals to, at least, 20 minutes or longer. Your stomach, mouth and brain are all connected and it takes 20 minutes of chewing before your stomach signals your brain that you are full. To feel full and successfully lose weight on any weight loss program, you need to eat slowly for 20 minutes or longer.

- Eat those spicy foods you enjoy. They increase your metabolic rate by 25%.

- Keep plenty of crunchy foods like raw vegetables and air-popped fat-free popcorn on hand. They're high in fibre, satisfying and filling.

- Avoid finger foods that are easy to eat in large amounts.

- Consume nuts only in small portions, as they are composed of up to 50% fat and have a high calorie count

- Make the kitchen off-limits at any time other than mealtime.

- Don't eat unnecessary foods. You don't need "all the fixings". Serve yourself normal portions of food. Three ounces of meat or a half cup of rice are plenty in one meal.

- Don't nibble on things throughout the day. Some treats have hundreds of calories.

- Start using a smaller plate for dinner. You'll feel like you ate more than you did.

- Don't work while eating. Separate all of your activities from your meals, so you can concentrate on what and how much you're eating.

- Don't eat a single bite of food while preparing meals. Use the **Slim & Sassy Chewing our Slim & Sassy Gum, it helps to cut the cravings.**

- Learn to control yourself at social affairs. Don't use them as an excuse to pig out.

- Always eat at the table, never in front of the TV set or with the radio on. You won't be able to monitor your eating habit when you're enjoying something else.

- Don't gulp. Savor each bite and concentrate on chewing every mouthful of food slowly.

- If you're a late-night eater, eat high fibre carbs such as a slice of brown bread or wholemeal cracker biscuit before bedtime to cut down on cravings and abdominal bulges.

- If tempted by a treat, you could eat half then give the rest away.

- Eat hot meals rather than cold. Your metabolism speeds up very slightly when you eat and again, if the food is hot.

- Don't eat anything for the last three or four hours of your day. Once you've had dinner, be done for the night.

- **Use the Metabolic Blend chewing gum between meals to help with chavings**.

- Be strong. You are in control of getting you from obese to slim, fit and sassy.

Use Motivate CPTG Essential Oil to Keep You Encouraged

- Get a bottle of Motivate CPTG Essential Oil and use throughout your journey.

- Weight loss is easier with a friend. Caring people can help motivate each other succeed.

- Don't weigh yourself too often. Use the tape measure and the fit of your clothes to monitor weight loss progress. Your weight fluctuates constantly and you can weigh more at night than you did in the morning.

- Never get seconds. Make a habit of stopping after one plate of food.

- Put leftovers away immediately to avoid further grazing.

- Read labels carefully. Some low fat items are very high in calories.

- To slow yourself down, eat with the opposite hand you usually eat with.

Stop the Cravings Using . ....

- Chew the Matabolic Gum. It speeds up the digestive system, burning more calories, and kills the craving. Metabolic blend in your liquids and use the TrimShakes.

- Craving chocolate? Eat a banana. It sometimes satisfies the yearning for chocolate and is much less fattening.

- Use the Metabolic Blend to curb the creavings.

- Use the TrimShakes help curb cravings.

Exercise Plays A Big Role In Weight Loss

- Exercise – even in school! Take advantage of the gym and PE classes in school. Participate in any sports.

- Spend at least 10 minutes per day exercising in your room.

- If possible, walk places instead of riding a car. You can even enjoy the scenic spots you will see as you walk.

- Use stairs instead of elevators if it's just a matter of 3-4 storeys.

- Limit your Social Media, TV and game times to 2 hours or less per day.

- Eat first before strolling at the mall with friends or alone. This way, calories will start burning and at the same time, you won't be tempted to order another burger or french fries or fast foods.

- Substitute activity for eating junk food. When the cravings hit, walk around the block, do some housework, read, or just do anything just that will take your mind off those old habits.

- Do at least thirty minutes of cardiovascular exercise, five days a week. This will condition you to burn fat more efficiently.

- Wear a pedometer if you can get one and see that you take 1,000 steps every day.

- If you have a sit-down job, get up every hour and walk around for five minutes or so.

- Dedicate two hours a week to weight training, concentrating on the larger muscles. Every other day is best.

What About Self-Esteem?

- The more positive your self-esteem, the better you feel about yourself, the faster and easier it will be for you to lose weight. When you are self-confident, you are better able to take charge of your life. Losing weight will help boost your positive self image.

- Negative emotions will also interfere with your weight loss program. It's difficult to stay motivated to lose weight when you feel bad. Over-reating often accompanies negative emotions such as depression, anxiety, fear, guilt and anger, hate, failures.

Thus, if you really want to lose weight and burn all the excess body fats away – to be physically fit and healthy – you have to deal with it properly. Proper plan, attitude, diet, exercise, and lifestyle comprise the proper way to achieve your goals. Success is not attained overnight so you have to really exert not just an effort, but also patience and determination, if you want to get slim, fit and sassy.

Don't shop when you're <u>hungry</u> you are setting yourself up for food failure. You'll only buy more fattening food. One big thing which might seem hard to do is to avoid people who constantly inviting you out to eat fast foods and indulge in over-eating. Another big set up for packing on the pounds especially around the stomach, legs and buttom is constant late night eating large meals with little time for digestion of food before sleep.

Why do you set yourself up to fail at losing weight? If you know there is the potential you will overeat, plan ahead to avoid the things that easily cause your weight gain. Most times, it's the wrong habits you have practiced overtime.

You are invited to start the 30-Day Lose Weight Plan and using the National appetite-coltrol Products and Supplements to curb the cravings and cut the fats.

Remember you are God's magificent creation and no man can reverse that. You must see yourself as a special treasure. Treat yourself as you would a special treasure chest. One to be filled with choice products that produces amazing results. You can do it. Get rid of your yesterday's behaviour and live strong in God starting today! He want to live in you too because you are His temple.

A WORD OF ENCOURAGEMENT TO THE OVERWEIGHT AND OBESE

Find Some Trusted Critics.

"*I believe that one of the greatest gifts that we can have in life are friends who love us enough to tell us the truth and risk our friendship to help us grow. We can always find people who, when we ask, will tell us what we want to hear. They will agree with us and tell us what we did well. I'm not saying that we don't want these people in our lives. We need them as well. But, when you are stuck, when you are falling behind on your dreams, and your strategies and efforts are not yielding the results you want, you better hope you have a friend that is willing to put it all on the line and be truthful because they love you. I will forever be grateful for those who figuratively grabbed me by the collar, shook me, and said, "Kyle, wake up! You are better than this. You can do more. You can be more.*"

Life has an incredible way of steering us toward the struggles that, when handled with grace, can turn us into the leaders that we need to become. You have an incredible power within you to get unstuck, to know that things will get better, and to know it can be handled. Don't ever quit when you're stuck, because those before you would tell you that the breakthrough is just on the other side and it is worth it." dōTERRA

Bonus # 6

Proper Personal Finance: Make Money With NAPS

Personal Finance and Free to Give

When talking about the financial state of US citizens, David Stirling, Founding Executive, CEO and President of dōTERRA says, "Our consumer debt today has exceeded what it was prior to the 2008 crash. We didn't learn a lot from our last recession, it appears. When I say consumer debt, I mean debt outside of mortgages or even car loans. It's credit card debt, or debt for things that aren't necessary like expensive furniture that add lots of little payments to bills each month." Considering that credit card debt in the US alone amounted to $712 billion in 2015, the importance of managing your finances and being aware of how you spend your money has never been more pressing if you want a secure financial future.

Debt might seem insurmountable if you're stuck with mounting bills, but it is a circumstance that you can change given some time and know-how.

You must first learn how to track your expenses to discover exactly where your money is going. This will take the most time: tracking your expenses for at least three months will help you get the full picture. Once you have three months of financial records in front of you, you must then ask yourself two questions. Look at each expense and ask:

1. Does this purchase make my life better?

2. Is there a more cost-effective alternative that provides the same benefit?

You likely will find ways that you can improve your financial situation, just by changing a few of your habits. Perhaps you need to make some bigger changes, like a car that has better fuel economy, or to figure out what you can take out of your grocery bills. Or, maybe make a lifestyle change to eat out less and make more homemade meals.

You will quickly discover that maybe you didn't need as much money as you thought to have the life you want. Putting money in savings could be just as big of a thrill as purchasing that new entertainment system.

If you truly want to make a change but need some help, <u>Free to Give</u>, a doTERRA-sponsored incentive program, could be that extra push that you need. Click on the link provided to find out more and enroll. You will also find helpful resources on the site, such as a free monthly budget, an expense tracker, and a debt payment tracker.

BONUS # 7

PROPER PRODUCTS TO MOTIVATE, CHEER, INCREASE PASSION, FORGIVE, CONSOLE, INCREASE PEACE

Featured on the Facebook page of Dr. David K. Hill

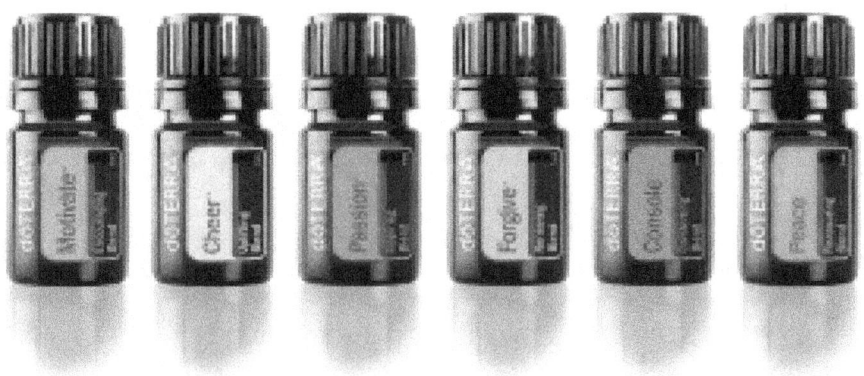

Have you ever wondered why a simple smell can provoke a strong emotion or trigger a specific memory? I know the smell of fresh homemade bread reminds me of my sweet mother. The dōTERRA Emotional Aromatherapy™ Kit is the perfect example of this, and here's why it works so well:

Essential oils are simply a mixture of volatile aromatic compounds. These compounds interact with the olfactory (smell) receptors in the nose. Our sense of smell can have a profound effect on our emotions, and simply inhaling the aroma can elicit an emotional response. The smell receptors located on the upper surface of the nasal cavity make direct links with the limbic system of the brain, where the scent is perceived and processed.

EMOTIONAL AROMATHERAPY SYSTEM

A revolutionary organization of aromatic plant families around a continuum of emotions for a simple, profound approach to using fragrant essential oils in emotional aromatherapy applications. Individual essential oils can be used with great effectiveness by skilled aromatherapists. This new kit makes emotional aromatherapy easy and accessible for anyone dealing with common negative emotions with a new line of proprietary essential oil blends representing six categories of emotional well-being.

Each delicate blend contains pure, therapeutic-grade essential oils that can be used aromatically or topically to help balance and brighten your changing moods. Just a few drops of these naturally complex, fragrant blends can elicit profound emotional responses to help you let go of burdens, find comfort and encouragement, or inspire you to dream with passion again.

Directions:

- Use aromatically in an essential oil diffuser.
- Apply 1-2 drops in your palms, rub hands together, cup in front of your nose, and inhale deeply.
- Dilute and apply topically to aromatherapy touch points such as the back of the neck, on the wrists, and over the heart.

Kit Contents:

1. **MOTIVATE: Encouraging Blend**. Are you frustrated at work? Do you have setbacks despite your best efforts, yet your confidence is still shaken? Or has misplaced trust left you cynical more often that your best self should be? Then stop, reset, and restart with Motivate Encouraging Blend of mint and citrus essential oils. Motivate

will help you unleash your creative powers and find the courage that comes from believing in yourself again. Go ahead and raise the bar—you can do it!

2. **CHEER**: **Uplifting Blend**. Everyone knows a bright disposition and cheerful attitude can smooth over many of the bumps and challenges of life, right? But, sometimes no amount of positive self-talk is enough to avoid the blues. Cheer Uplifting Blend of citrus and spice essential oils provides a cheerful boost of happiness and positivity when you are feeling down. Its sunshiny, fresh, optimistic aroma will brighten any moment of your day.

3. **PASSION**: **Inspiring Blend**. Have you lost your why, your mojo, your passion? Too much of even a good thing can become predictable and boring over time. Passion Inspiring Blend of spice and herb essential oils will help you rekindle excitement in your life. Jump out of an airplane, dive into an ocean, or try something scary like dancing. With Passion, you will find the daring to try something new, as wells as discover renewed joy for the current blessings in your life.

4. **FORGIVE**: **Renewing Blend**. Are you carrying a burden that grows heavier with time? Would you be better off just letting it go and facing a future unfettered by anger and guilt? When you are ready to move forward, Forgive Renewing Blend of tree and herb essential oils will help you discover the liberating action of forgiving, forgetting, and moving on. Start each of your tomorrows relieved and contented with Forgive Renewing Blend.

5. **CONSOLE**: **Comforting Blend**. Losing something or someone you love can be deeply disorienting and painful. Words unspoken and questions unanswered may keep you worried and unsettled. Console Comforting Blend of floral and tree essential oils will help you close the door on sadness and take your first steps on a

hopeful path toward emotional healing. Bind your broken heart with Console Comforting Blend.

6. <u>**PEACE**</u>: **Reassuring Blend**. Are life's anxious moments leaving you feeling overwhelmed and afraid? Peace Reassuring Blend of floral and mint essential oils is a positive reminder you don't have to be perfect to find peace. Slow down, take a deep breath, and reconnect with the composed, collected you. Everything turning out fine begins with believing it will—and a few drops of Peace Reassuring Blend.

If you are struggling with accomplishing your goal to lose weight everyday.

These aromata uplifting CPTG Certified Pure Therapeutic Grade® Essential Oils will uplift, motivate, cheer you along, so your passion will be present. Your heart will be at peace as you forgive the people who hurt you in the past causing food addiction to start. Console yourself in the fact that you are now on your way to reinvent yourself.

TO PURCHASE THIS KIT TO MOTIVATE YOURSELF TO LOSE WEIGHT

<u>**CLICK HERE AND GET THE MEMBERSHIP FIRST TO GET 25% OFF THE COST.**</u>

BENEFITS OF dōTERRA MEMBERSHIP

<u>**Free to Give**</u>,

Financial Freedom is Attainable

Free to Give is a new dōTERRA-sponsored incentive program designed to inspire Wellness Advocates to pay off debt and live abundantly while becoming free financially to be in a better position to give to others.

"dōTERRA wants to be known as the company that helps the most people get out of debt." – Corey Lindley, Founding Executive, Chief Financial Officer dōTERRA International

ENROLL IN THE FREE TO GIVE PROGRAM

Focus on Four Types of Debt

Being financially free is a long-term goal for most people. With the Free to Give program, Wellness Advocates will see the benefits that come from being free of debt and loans, allowing you to enjoy living with financial freedom. In doing so, you will be able to give to others who have just started their own financial independence journey.

We have categorized the most common kinds of debt into four categories:

1. Credit Cards   Car Payments
2. Loans and Medical Bills   Mortgage

Paying off any one of these debt categories is a huge accomplishment. Each Wellness Advocate enrolled in the Free to Give program who achieves financial independence in any one of these areas will receive a token to symbolize this achievement. Our goal is that our Wellness Advocates can begin the journey to becoming free one category at a time, until you are ultimately in a place where you are Free to Give.

Becoming a Wellness Advocate

Wholesale Membership

doTERRA® offers product through a yearly wholesale membership. For a low membership fee of $35.00, a Wellness Advocate will be able to purchase products at wholesale prices 25 percent below retail.

Renewal Fee

After becoming a Wellness Advocate, the yearly renewal fee for a wholesale membership is $25.00. This renewal fee comes with a free bottle of Peppermint, one of the most popular oils doTERRA offers, a retail value of $27.33.

CONCLUSION OF HOW TO LOSE WEIGHT EVERYDAY USING NAPS & LUCK

So you think you're ready to lose weight and burn fats? To motivate you more, actually, it's not just your heavy weight and your stubborn body fats that you can eliminate with these proper NAPS solutions and guidelines; but also a really dangerous illness that could lead you to your grave—obesity.

Obesity is a killer and by 2030 it promises to become a pandemic per the World Health Organization (WHO). Do you know what that means to your life and mine? It means we have to help everyone to learn how to care for their bodies properly to be able to live longer, and look younger. To be slim, fit and sassy. To trust in God more and ask him to bless with boldness and confidence. For God to give BIG will-power to go do what he wants of us.

If we do not hurry up and get this critical information plus these Natural Apptetite-control Products & Supplements out into the hands of overweight people, obesity will cause only harm to innocent people. It's worse than criminals that try to attack us. My TV news announce some of the bad people to make me aware. My local police dropped off flyers when crimals are seen and known in the surroundings. They can always be avoided and fight against when encountered. There are powerful authorities that publish their faces when caught, and give enough punishment according to how badly they behaved. But obesity is far different from lawbreakers. Although both may kill us, obesity kills without the victim knowing it. I have seen many patients lose a limb and still complaining of the **phantom pain** of what feels like it's coming from the body part that's no longer there.

Obesity poisons both our body and mind. For the former, it's weapon is an overload of fats targetting essential body parts and organs; thus, bringing serious complications like heart diseases, cancer, liver, kidney and stomach problems, plus a lot more. As for the latter, negative thoughts are what it uses, making the victim feel inferior and underrated, developing such poor self-esteem.

It is terrible to see even the very young people so overweight and obese. They are burdened down with bills of providing new clothes every few months to cover their buldging fats. Yet they fail to make the adjustments in diet and activity. They seek out friends who will accompany them to binge out on sugary drinks, salty and fatty foods. Isn't it very sad?

So before it becomes too late, before obesity attacks us and bring us all down to our last breath, why don't we attack obesity directly where it hurts most—in the taste buds and activity center of life? Let us kill obesity first before it kills us all. We must make the choice in our mind to quit the excuse lifestyle. We will never kill this BIG obesity by ourselves. So, its time to call in the BIG guys. Oh it is Jesus, His Father God and The Holy Spirit.

Perhaps that is the reason why the world has no place for obesity – because it kills. Well then, show the world that you can kill what they have been rejecting all the while. Let them notice you, see you, and recognize you the way you really should be—slim, fit and sassy. Congratulations!

SUMMARYOF HOW TO LOSE WEIGHT EVERYDAY

Overweight and Obesity are Killers. Call In the big Guns

Overweight and obesity are killers and you are no match to fight them alone. It is time to call in the BIG powerful guys with the BIG guns. It is an army of three-in-one. It is Jesus, His Holy Father—God, and The Holy Spirit!

Stop Depending on Yourself Alone

We may not be powerful alone to control overweight and obesity, or even the foods we become addicted to. But when we call in the BIG guys from above and they take over, we are assured of this one promise, no weight can hold our bodies down. They will help us deal with the issues we face daily that led to overeating and lack of frequent exercising. God's peace will be in our hearts and that is sufficient to calm us down. His grace is sufficient so give him the glory.

There are two kinds of weights we would like us all to lose and they are:

1. **Weights that are made of fats**. These kinds become plaque that blocks and clog our arteries causing heart attacks—the number one killer of humans today.
2. **The second weight is the issues of the mind and heart** that so easily derail and set us back. These are emotions like, fear, doubts, sadness, anger, hatred, malice, envy, fightings among ourselves, obedience to satanic voices and using his devices.

To determine which category of physical weight group you belong in, go to the accompanying website, http://lose-weight-everyday.com// :and use the BMI Calculator to determine your level of fat based on the common height-weight relationship and through our body mass index (BMI). Either way, one has to know if he is healthy or not in order to make certain adjustments, or even worse, determine if we need treatment.

In the Introduction Section of this book, are the eleven Natural Appetite-control Products & Supplements that are helping millions of people to reinvent their lives. If you are broken physically, there are products to support and maintain your body. If you are broke financially, you can get the membeship then encourage people to sample the various products based on their health deviations—from abuse, acne to weight and wrinkles. I bet you this one thing, many of these hurting people, will want to use the NAPS and CPTG Certified Pure Therapeutic Grade® Essential oils to uplift, energerize and help their broken bodies. That right there is now you start your home business. You will become victorious through your difficulties.

Obesity, defines as being 20 percent or more above one's desirable weight range, is a serious illness that should not be left untreated so as not to bring serious addiction, heath and wealth complications into your life, jumpstart your life today using NAPS. According to studies, obesity may be caused by genetic factors, i.e. if any of the family members, especially the parents, suffers from such sickness, the children will most likely receive it from them. Improper eating habits and/or lifestyle failures along with doubts, fears and lack of trust.

Effects of obesity include both psychological and biological aspects like heart diseases, cancer, diabetes, and much more. Thus, if obesity can't be stopped immediately, who knows what could happen next? Ending of one's life is not impossible, you know many are ending their lives using their knives, spoons and forks.

Untreated, obesity will lead to a slow death. To think that I use my own knife, fork, and spoon to dig my very own grave? How foolish!

I have cared for many such foolish patients from the Emergency Room to the Intensive Care Unit, Vascular Unit more. All I see and hear about are the complications of obesity overwhelmed bodies and ruined dreams and lives. People who cannot walk anymore therefore, cannot attend children or grandchildren graduations, weddings, or special family events. Instead, they are hooked up to breathing machines in the hospitals begging for pain pills that barly take their physical pains away.

My biggest job in the hospital, community and online right now is to educate everyone so they know that simple changes in diet, lifestyle and habits could save much suffering and event prevent further deterioration of their bodies. Unfortunately for many, diets do not work to lose weight and keep it off. So something has to work and that's why this book was created. It comes with the eleven (11) Natural Appetite-control Products & Supplements for losing the weights. There are products for addiction, fear, lack of motivation, overweight and obesity, plus so much more. Yes, finally, it is your turn to lose weight naturally and keep it off.

My only mission is to prevent your suffering. There is a survey of 188 countries that shows that nearly 30 percent of the global population, or 2.1 billion people, are either overweight or obese. Not a single country has lowered its obesity rate since 1980, the first of its kind study showed.

Perhaps most troubling, kids are heavier than ever, the survey by the Institute for Health Metrics and Evaluation (IHME) at the University of Washington finds. The percentage of overweight or obese children and teenagers has increased by nearly 50 percent since 1980 and now more than 22 percent of girls and nearly 24 percent of boys in developed countries are overweight or obese."

Luckily, it's not yet too late. Obesity, indeed, can be be cured…and even prevented. All it takes is a "proper" way of dealing with it. It needs NAPS, dependence on Christ for help, obedience to God to live in moderation, plus patience, determination, and the will to succceed. And before you know it, your weight might have decreased by 20 pounds or your waistline have been trimmed down by 10 inches. Isn't that cool? Not to mention, healthy and poverty prevention from savings of copays, surgery bills, cancer treatments and your happiness!

The Proper Way to Lose Weight Everyday

The proper way is actually just your everyday living and habits only done properly. First, you got to have a proper plan. This includes setting a goal of what you want to happen and accomplish in a certain period of time. It should be definite and realistic. Managing your plan in an organized manner is the critical part of the plan.

Time and duration of activities to be done throughout the day or week should be taken note and remembered. Positive thinking and right attitude towards the weights are also important in making all plans work effectively. Believing in something to happen triggers the body to do things that could make your hopes and dreams come true. The brain frinds the way to make things happen that we think about. Thus, although plans are still on the mind and not yet turning into reality, they are a good help in starting to make things happen. Speak success into your situations.

Eating is the habit most associated with body weight and obesity. Everyone eats...but not everyone does it properly. Proper diet should contain all food nutrients such as carbohydrates, proteins, vitamins, and minerals, making your meal healthy and nutritious. In contrast to what most people believe, all fats are not bad for our body. In fact, there are good ones, the unsaturated fats in which their intake should not be limited. The unhealthy fats are those that belong to the saturated group of fats. All the NAPS products are CPTG Certified. More than organic and 100% pure.

Since obesity is related to heavier weight and excess body fats, weight loss with regards to food intake involves either one of the two ways: eating low-fat foods, or consuming fat-burner foods. The former diet is about substituting low-fat foods with those with high fat contents, while the latter refers to simply eating foods that burn excess fats in the body. Any of the said diets will surely help you lose weight and get rid of those difficult to lose body fats.

As I staed earlier on in this book, losing weight is not dependent on right diet alone. To speed it up and burn more calories faster, one should engage on proper exercises and these include deep breathing, walking, aerobic exercises, cardiovaslcular exercises, and weight training. Also, there are exercise machines and tools that can help lose weight such as treadmill, exercise bikes, steppers, and many more. Plus the NAPS supplements.

Lastly, if you really want to stop overweight and obesity, one must check and watch the lifestyle, maintain the body with NAPS, Live Uner Christ Knowledge—acronymed LUCK. To change from improper lifestyle, is comprised of simple and little everyday things, that will add up over time in losing weight. It also involved practices and beliefs that stop the negative thoughts and practices. So instead of fear, hate sadness etc and turning to foods and drinks for satisfaction, you start some activity but seek God's help to exercie and not be tired or quit.. Alsways on guard for new habits as, one should not take his habits for granted even those that are as trivial as eating in front of the TV or whats the proper foods to eat and when.

APPENDIX A

Required Weight Ranges Based on Weight & Height

Males		Females	
HEIGHT	WEIGHT	HEIGHT	WEIGHT
5'4"	117 - 163	5'0"	96 - 138
5'5"	120 - 167	5'1"	99 - 141
5'6"	124 - 173	5'2"	102 - 144
5'7"	128 - 178	5'3"	105 - 149
5'8"	132 - 183	5'4"	108 - 152
5'9"	136 - 187	5'5"	111 - 156
5'10"	140 - 193	5'6"	114 - 161
5'11"	144 - 198	5'7"	118 - 165
6'0"	148 - 204	5'8"	122 - 169
6'1"	152 - 209	5'9"	126 - 174
6'2"	156 - 215	5'10"	130 - 179
6'3"	160 - 220	5'11"	134 - 185
6'4"	169 - 231	6'0"	138 - 190

APPENDIX B: Lose Weight Everyday Weekly Diary

Date:

Weight:

BMI:

Weekly Reflections:

Measurements:

Waist:

Hips:

Bust/Chest:

Right Thigh:

Left Thigh:

Right Arm:

Left Arm:

Weight Change This Week:

How Did I Feel About Myself This Week?

126

APPENDIX C

Calories Burned During Exercises
(and other activities)

ACTIVITY	CALORIES/HOUR
Bowling	250
Cleaning Windows	350
Cycling	400
Dancing	300
Football	450
Gardening	250
General Housework	190
Golf	250
Horse Riding	450
Ironing	250
Jogging	500
Mowing the Lawn	400
Running	900
Scrubbing Floors	275
Skiing	500
Swimming	500
Walking	250

RESOURCES USED OR MENTIONED

- See more at: https://doterra.com/US/en/blog/recipe-cucumber-avocado-open-faced-sandwiches#sthash.T6mpgO8B.dpuf

Tips: - See more at: https://doterra.com/US/en/blog/recipes-green-smoothie#sthash.O0GVbida.dpuf

https://doterra.com/US/en/pl/weight-management

4 Laws of Financial Prosperity include the book, *The 4 Laws of Financial Prosperity* ($11.99) and The Debt Down Tool ($14 for one year).

- See more at: https://doterra.com/US/en/blog/inspiration-personal-finance-and-free-to-give#sthash.3hlhSJcG.dpuf
- See more at: https://doterra.com/US/en/blog/sharing-becoming-elite#sthash.EFNQvDkJ.dpuf
See more at: https://doterra.com/US/en/blog/spotlight-doterra-motivate-encouraging-blend#sthash.nkEwuS6o.dpuf
See more at: https://doterra.com/US/en/blog/leader-ideas-9-ways-to-get-unstuck-in-your-business#sthash.VyZtbF9d.dpuf
- See more at: https://doterra.com/US/en/blog/science-wellness-emotional-aromatherapy#sthash.9TJ46OLC.dpuf
1. WHO. Physical status: the use and interpretation of anthropometry. Report of a WHO Expert Committee. WHO Technical Report Series 854. Geneva: World Health Organization, 1995.
2. WHO. Obesity: preventing and managing the global epidemic. Report of a WHO Consultation. WHO Technical Report Series 894. Geneva: World Health Organization, 2000.
3. WHO/IASO/IOTF. The Asia-Pacific perspective: redefining obesity and its treatment. Health Communications Australia: Melbourne, 2000.
4. James WPT, Chen C, Inoue S. Appropriate Asian body mass indices? Obesity Review, 2002; 3:139.
5. WHO expert consultation. Appropriate body-mass index for Asian populations and its implications for policy and intervention strategies. The Lancet, 2004; 157-163.
The U.S. Departments of Agriculture, Health and Human Services
Medline Plus
Self.com
KidsHealth

WRITE DOWN YOUR PLAN HOW TO

LOSE WEIGHT EVERYDAY HERE